Turning Points
in the Life
of a Fisherman

Turning Points

in the Life
of a Fisherman

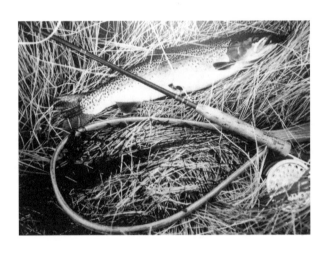

David Van Lear

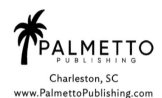

Charleston, SC
www.PalmettoPublishing.com

Turning Points in the Life of a Fisherman

First Edition

Hardcover ISBN: 979-8-88590-697-5
Paperback ISBN: 979-8-88590-698-2

David H. Van Lear, Ph.D.

David Van Lear is the Clemson University Robert A. Bowen Professor Emeritus of Forestry.

VAN LEAR ATTENDED HAMPDEN-SYDNEY College and Virginia Tech before completing his doctoral work at the University of Idaho and his postdoctoral work at the University of Florida. Van Lear is recognized as a leading authority on the silviculture and ecology of Southern pine and upland hardwood ecosystems.

During his long career, Van Lear was honored by the Society of American Foresters who named him a Fellow and presented him with the Barrington Moore Memorial Award. He also received the Outstanding Hardwood Research Award from the National Hardwood Lumber Association. Honors from his time at Clemson University include the Godley-Snell Award for excellence in agricultural research and Researcher of the Year from Sigma XI. The Association of Fire Ecology awarded Van Lear with the Lifetime Achievement Award, and the South Carolina Forestry Association presented him with the Charles Flory Award for his distinguished service. Van Lear was named Outstanding Alumnus of the College of Forest Resources at Virginia Tech. He was also recognized by Trout Unlimited with the Distinguished Service Award for his efforts in leading its stream and brook trout restoration efforts in South Carolina.

Dr. Van Lear and his wife Carolyn live in Clemson, South Carolina.

Read more of Van Lear's story in his previous book, *Memories Made and Lessons Learned During a Lifetime of Angling,* and online at *clemson.world/you-can-go-home/.*

Table of Contents

Chapter I

Turn Around!

As I approached Montrose, Colorado, a highway sign pointed the way to the Black Canyon of the Gunnison River. I was driving from Virginia to Yellowstone National Park for another fly-fishing "fix." I had fallen in love with Yellowstone National Park when I had worked there during five summers after high school graduation. Here is where I learned to fly fish and began a life-long addiction.

Naturally, given the opportunity in 1971, I headed back to Yellowstone. I had chosen a southern route so I could see and perhaps fish a couple of the beautiful streams in Colorado before reaching Yellowstone. I only had about 10 days before I would report to a new job at Clemson University, so time was short. When I reached Durango, Colorado, in the southwest corner of the state, I headed north on Route 550 toward Montrose.

The Black Canyon of the Gunnison River sounded like a place worth seeing. Maybe, I thought, I could fish the Gunnison River for half a day or so. The right turn I took outside of Montrose, Colorado, proved to be a real turning point — one of many — that helped determine the direction of my life.

That particular turn also almost cost me my life.

There must be a way down.

THE BLACK CANYON OF the Gunnison would be made a national park in 1999, but that was still 28 years in the future. Black Canyon was awesome — more impressive in some ways than the Grand Canyon of the Yellowstone, a canyon I was intimately familiar with from my summers spent working in the park. Several times I had hiked with friends into the Yellowstone canyon to fish for cutthroat trout during the salmonfly hatch, and not once did I feel in danger of falling. I had to be careful, yes, but I had not been in imminent danger.

On this Sunday morning as I drove along the north rim, the Black Canyon of the Gunnison had a different feel from the bright and beautiful canyon of Yellowstone that I was so familiar with. The Black Canyon felt deeper, darker and narrower. It seemed more dangerous and foreboding, and most important of all, there did not appear to be any reasonable way to access the river I saw far below.

As I walked along the rim of the canyon, I noticed a small sign that read "Good Trout Fishing 2,000 Feet Below." It didn't say anything about how to get down there, and I didn't see any trails leading to the river. How could I access the river?

Since no one was around on that quiet, rather lonely, morning who could answer that question for me, I started looking around for myself. Surely one of the many ravines, or washes, that fell sharply off the rim would lead an angler down to the river. Why would there be a sign advertising the trout fishing down in the canyon if there was no way to get down there?

Several of the ravines appeared to lead at least halfway down to the river, but from the rim it was impossible to see beyond those inflection points. Being a young bachelor at the time, without anyone to reprimand me for being so stupid, I decided to give the most promising of those ravines a try. I put on my waders, laced on my hiking boots, grabbed my fly rod and fishing vest, and started climbing and sliding on my rear end down the ravine.

What a brainless decision that was! After I had climbed and slid about halfway down to the river, the ravine suddenly gave way to an almost-vertical drop of at least 1,000 feet. I was just one step from eternity!

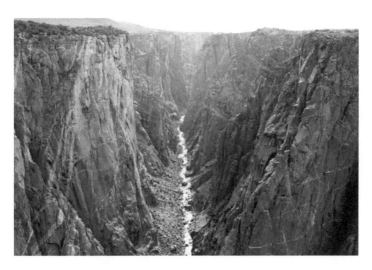

The Black Canyon of the Gunnison, a canyon where I climbed and slid halfway to the river below before being forced to turn back by a 1,000-foot vertical drop.

"Good grief!" I yelled (or something like that), as I struggled to stabilize my position to avoid sliding over the brink. Catching my breath, I realized what a foolish idea this had been. If I had gone another foot, I would have slid off into nothing and fallen to my death.

No one would have known where I was. I hadn't told anyone of my stupid idea to access the Gunnison River by climbing down into the canyon. In my mind, I pictured a fisherman or floater one day discovering a scavenger-ravaged body and wondered how it got there. "Surely not from above," they would think. "Only a fool would attempt to climb down that cliff!"

Gathering my wits, I carefully reversed direction and slowly, on hands and knees, crawled up and out of the ravine. As far as I know, no one saw this brilliant show of stupidity.

A life of addiction

I readily admit an addiction to fly fishing. And sometimes I have wondered about this particular addiction. Am I sane? Is this addiction so deeply ingrained in my being that I cannot make rational decisions? Looking back on the Black Canyon experience, I know I learned a lesson, but it could have been my final lesson. What a dangerous risk I took just to fly fish in that river!

In other aspects of my life, I think I make fairly normal decisions, including some great decisions, like marrying my wife Carolyn, but with fly fishing, I have often wondered how sound my decisions were.

That Sunday morning, I was able to get back in my truck and travel on to Yellowstone, where grizzly bears were the only things I had to worry about. This time, I escaped unscathed. But in the 50 years since that experience at the Black Canyon of the Gunnison, I have had a number of other adventures, some dangerous, some challenging, some rewarding. At 81 years old, I realize that my life has been shaped by a succession of decisions, turning points that together made me the person I became, no matter how flawed that may be. Today, I understand how a different decision at these points could have changed my path and made me a completely different kind of person.

I don't want to imply that I turned out to be a great person; far from that. But I believe that the story of a good person who started life with a little ambition, overcame difficulties, and through hard work, persistence, good fortune, and with a lot of help from family, friends and a "good" addiction — to fly fishing — is a story worth telling. I think I turned out to be a pretty successful person. At the least I am someone who is happy with how his life turned out.

I am telling my story for two reasons. The first is a purely selfish one. I want to recall my life before my memory makes these recollections difficult or impossible. It almost seems that I was blessed throughout my life to have been given opportunities that molded me, opportunities that often happened without any encouragement from me. Whether blessed or just lucky, I will say that once these opportunities presented themselves, I worked hard to bring them to fruition. I have had an interesting life full of joy, sadness, adventures and opportunities that have taken me from the Allegheny Mountains of Virginia to a chaired professorship at Clemson University. Along the way, I have been fortunate to benefit from major turning points that had a profound influence on my life.

Second, my story includes dealing with the effects of the common but often overlooked disorders of depression and/or bipolar disorder.

Perhaps my story will help inspire a young person who starts out in life much like I did, without any major aspirations but who wants to make a success of his or her life, perhaps not so much from the standpoint of making a lot of money, but just in knowing that they did their best, were morally good, empathized with others and were respected by peers.

Chapter 2

Growing Up and Dealing with Cyclothymia

I HAVE ALWAYS FELT, from the time I was a college student, that I had a mild degree of bipolar disorder, which is called cyclothymia. What made me think I had, and probably still have, cyclothymia?

For decades I have had so many of the symptoms of the disorder that I have self-diagnosed my behavior. In addition, bipolar disorder tends to be hereditary, and it runs deep in my family. I have experienced many of these symptoms such as excessive activity, extreme happiness followed by periods of sadness, the need to achieve or over-achieve, anxiety and even times of risky behavior such as that climb over a cliff to reach the Gunnison River. However, I have not experienced all the symptoms of cyclothymia. For example, though "talking more than usual," is listed as an indication of the disease, I have always been a fairly quiet person.

Certainly, most people will say they have high and low feelings, or other of these symptoms, but I believe they have haunted me to a greater degree than for most folks.

CYCLOTHYMIA

Cyclothymia is defined by the American Psychological Association as "a mood disorder characterized by periods of hypomanic symptoms and periods of depressive symptoms." The Mayo Clinic describes it as "emotional ups and downs ... not as extreme as those in bipolar I or II disorder" and lists the symptoms as:

- An exaggerated feeling of happiness or well-being
- Extreme optimism
- Inflated self-esteem
- Talking more than usual
- Poor judgment that can result in risky behavior or unwise choices
- Racing thoughts
- Irritable or agitated behavior
- Excessive physical activity
- Increased drive to perform or achieve goals
- Decreased need for sleep
- Tendency to be easily distracted
- Inability to concentrate

Sources: *https://dictionary.apa.org/major-depressive-episode* and *https://www.mayoclinic.org/diseases-conditions/cyclothymia/diagnosis-treatment/drc-20371281*

FORTUNATELY FOR ME, I have been able, since I started college, to utilize my hypomanic symptoms (symptoms less severe than those of bipolar disorder I and II) to be productive and function at a high level. For example, when I became overly anxious about making professional presentations, something I did hundreds of times throughout my career, I would use the anxious feeling to push me to be well-prepared for the task and thereby able to do a good job, perhaps even an outstanding job, in my mind. It worked for me. In general, I would over-prepare, work harder, put in more hours. Whatever I needed to do to succeed, I did.

Others in my family also suffered from the effects of bipolar disease with differing outcomes. Fortunately for me, I was able to use cyclothymia to my advantage. It allowed me to be highly productive when I was having mild hypomanic episodes, and when I felt sad and depressed, rather than using drugs or alcohol, I used fly fishing and thoughts of my generally happy life to lift my spirits.

It's all true

THIS IS A TRUE story. I inherited my mom's need to be honest, so what I am relating here is the truth, with perhaps just a little exaggeration — fishermen can't help it. However, since so much of my story involves fishing, I must say that since 1984, I have kept fishing journals in which I recorded each of my fishing trips: where I fished, weather and water conditions, hatches, flies I used, who I fished with and how efficient I was, i.e., the number of fish caught per hour of fishing. It's been fun for me to occasionally go back to my journals and reminisce about those many fishing trips over the decades. They also kept me honest and occasionally helped me understand how the fish of some fishermen — not mine, of course — can keep growing long after they were caught. I must admit that some of my catches may have grown a little bit, too. So, a fishing journal keeps us all honest.

Fortunately, I have pictures to back up most of my fish stories, and I have awards to back up my career accomplishments. This will be the true story of how I progressed from that hillbilly in the mountains of Virginia to a successful chaired professor of forestry at Clemson University.

Life in Clifton Forge

I WAS BORN ON December 1, 1940, in Clifton Forge, a small town of about 5,000 people in the Allegheny Mountains of Virginia. Clifton Forge sat alongside the Jackson River, now a fishable river downstream of Covington, Virginia, but badly polluted by effluent from the West Virginia Pulp and Paper Company when I was growing up. In those days, the river below Covington ran black and smelled bad — no fishing for me, unfortunately, in that river.

However, there was another river, the Cowpasture River, that was just a short distance away. The Cowpasture, about the same size as the Jackson, is one of the most beautiful and unpolluted rivers in Virginia. It is the river where I learned to fish, which became a hobby and eventually the addiction that I believe helped shape the direction of my life.

I had what I'd consider to be a fairly normal childhood, sometimes happy and sometimes sad. I am not really sure what brought about the feelings of sadness, but whatever it was, these sad times were never so serious that I considered seeing a doctor about them, and the feelings would come and go. What made me the happiest was having a loving family and fishing, which has been a constant since I was about 12 years old.

As I mentioned earlier, my mood swings may have occurred because of a predisposition toward bipolar disorder, a disease that ran deep on my dad's side of the family. While I was never diagnosed with the disease, I definitely had symptoms, such as periods of sadness, as well as times of highs when I thought I could do about anything I set my mind to. In any event, fishing helped me through the sad times and hard work, endurance and fear of failure helped me be highly productive during hypomanic times. I believed my symptoms were so mild that I could handle them without any medical assistance. Perhaps a psychiatrist might have said that I didn't have this condition, but as the old saying goes, "If it walks like a duck and quacks like a duck, then it is a duck." I think I had and still have cyclothymia.

When I was very young — up to about age four — my dad, Edward Harper Van Lear, worked as manager of the meat department for Kroger, a large chain grocery store in my hometown. My mom, Catherine Hyde Van Lear, was a stay-at-home housewife who cared for me and my brother, Edward "Eddie" Tillman, who was three years older than me, and my younger sister Mary Kathryn "Kitty." Even though Mom, at about age 12, had suffered from rheumatic fever which left her with a rheumatic heart, she was a very sweet woman who never complained about her health.

Dad was a hard worker and a good father. Dad was very active in the Clifton Forge community. And he was an alcoholic.

Dad had not been a star student by any means in school, but he was a born leader. He was president of his freshman and sophomore classes at the University of Richmond, but he dropped out of school in 1929 after his sophomore year, at the beginning of the Great Depression. Times were hard, and his family did not have the financial resources for him to continue his college education. Considering that the country was in the midst of the depression, Dad was lucky to be hired by the local Kroger store after he dropped out of college.

In 1944, my dad was offered a better job as the manager of the meat department of a larger Kroger store in Bristol, Tennessee, where we moved and where my sister, Kitty, was born. But he soon tired of working for the large chain and moved the family back to Clifton Forge, where he and his brother-in-law, Fred Hall, who had been manager of the produce department at Kroger, went into business for themselves. They opened a small grocery store just across the street from the Kroger store where they had previously worked.

They named their store The Food Center, and it was a bustling little business. However, the partnership didn't last long, and Dad bought Uncle Fred out after only a few years. Dad and The Food Center continued to hold their own against the big chain store across the street for more than two decades.

To me, my father and mother were wonderful parents, although my dad was a closet alcoholic and, I believe, had undiagnosed bipolar disorder. Doctors in Clifton Forge didn't know much about mental illness in those days. I believe that Dad drank to help him handle the periodic depressions that his bipolar condition caused.

Dad was never mean or abusive to my mom or us children. He loved all of us and never laid a hand, in anger, on any of us — not even a little spank on our rear ends. Dad had a strong deep voice, and all he had to do to get our undivided attention was to speak firmly to us.

Dad was well respected in Clifton Forge and ran a healthy business at his small grocery store for about 25 years. He was an extremely hard worker, never missing a day of work. He couldn't afford to. He would have worried about who was minding his store. Dad offered a couple of specialties that none of the larger chain grocery stores in town, like Kroger and A&P, could claim. His store delivered groceries to people, especially the elderly and disabled, who couldn't get downtown to buy their own, and he let customers buy their groceries on credit. They could call in their orders, store clerks would fill them, and Dad would have his driver deliver them all over town.

Often, I was part of that delivery team. I remember working at Dad's store on some Saturdays in high school when we — I was the assistant truck driver then — would deliver between 100 and 150 orders all over town. This was in addition to his in-store business — a healthy business indeed.

Dad was president of the Methodist Men's Bible Class for a number of years when I was in high school and brought record numbers of men to his Sunday school class. One Sunday, 310 men showed up for Sunday school, a gathering so large that they had to meet in the church sanctuary. They didn't come to hear Dad preach. He just kept things light and lively and got important people, including state politicians such as J. Lindsay Almond, the Virginia attorney general who would later become governor, to come speak to the class.

Dad often recruited men to come to Sunday school by calling them in the evening during the week, asking them to come to Sunday's class and, as I remember him saying, "Bring a friend."

Dad was not a strongly religious man. He was a Christian, but I think he viewed being president of the men's Bible class as good for his business. After all, his store was only a half block from the Methodist Church. In fact, when he began to think he wasn't getting as much business from members of that church as he thought he should, he switched his membership to the Presbyterian Church and soon became president of their men's Bible class. Dad was definitely a born leader and a shrewd businessman, too.

I remember him working late into the night on his tax returns as the April 15th deadline was approaching, or on half-page ads for the local newspaper advertising his store's produce and meat products. He was one hard-working man, and I was so proud of him. It was also Dad who taught me how to fish and to love fishing.

Our close family unit also included a dog that Dad got for us in 1952. He was a little chow-shepherd mix about eight weeks old, that we named him Sparky. Sparky went on hikes in the woods with my brother and me, and would swim in the river with us. He would even let Dad playfully squeeze his paw until he yipped while we were watching TV. It must not have hurt Sparky because he would always go back for more.

Sparky was the most loving and loyal dog a family could ask for, and we all loved him in return. He played a central part in our family happiness.

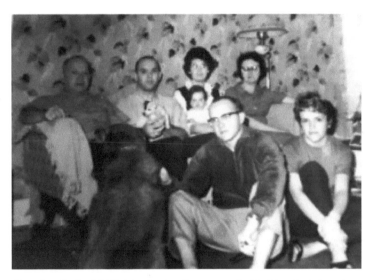

Our family in 1965 (clockwise from top left): My dad, brother
Eddy and his wife Lillian and baby Edward, my mom, my
sister Kitty, me and Sparky

As far as I was concerned, Dad's only fault was his alcoholism.

Frequently, after a hard day's work at his store, and maybe during
work, he would take a few, or more, snorts from the bottle of Jack
Daniels or Jim Beam that he hid in the bathroom of his store. Then
he would come home, not drunk, but "high," eat supper that Mom
had prepared for him. In the summer, he would work for a couple of
more hours in his garden or cut the grass on his John Deere mower.
If he didn't have something he wanted to do in the yard or garden, he
would sit down in his easy chair and fall asleep within minutes. Then
he would wake up, watch the 11 o'clock news and go to bed. Dad was
an unbelievably hard worker and had outstanding endurance.

Only once do I remember us being so worried about his drinking
that it almost caused us to panic. That night, Dad did not come home

after work. As the hours went by, we began to really worry. Was he all right? Our phone calls to his store went unanswered. Finally, Mom, Eddy and I went to his store and peered through the windows. It was dark inside, but we finally were able to make out Dad's body lying on top of the checkout counter. Was he dead or alive?

The three of us were eventually able to make enough noise banging on the windows to wake him up. He had taken a drink or two too many and decided to take a nap on the countertop. When Dad came to the door and rather sheepishly let us in, it was about 10 p.m. We were all just thankful that he was alive, if just a little bit drunk.

Despite his alcoholism, Dad was amazingly healthy, and he never missed a day of work from sickness in his whole working career until the last weeks of his life. I don't remember him ever having even the common cold. However, in 1974 when he was 65 years old, he had to go into the hospital for a hernia operation from which he never fully recovered.

After his hernia operation, Dad quit drinking. Within a couple weeks after the operation, he became depressed and couldn't manage his business or make sound decisions. When he was drinking, alcohol must have allowed Dad to function through what I believe was his bipolar disorder.

In November of that year, I was an associate professor at Clemson University. Mom called me and asked if I could come home and be with Dad for a few days to encourage him and help get him back on his feet. She was really worried about him.

So, I went home and went to the store with Dad for several days, trying to cheer him up and offer up any help I could. Finally, I told Mom that I had to go back to Clemson, but I told her to call me if she needed me to come back. I didn't have a good feeling about leaving.

A week later, I was attending a forestry conference in Charleston, South Carolina, when I heard an announcement over the loudspeaker that I had an emergency call at the front desk.

When I picked up the phone, it was my brother Eddy saying, "Dave, Dad is dead. He shot himself."

The impact of those words almost floored me. As I stood there by the front desk, head sagging, my department head, Robert Allen, walked over to me. He had heard the hotel paging me to the phone. I had told Dr. Allen before I left for the Charleston meeting that Dad was deeply in debt because many of his customers were abusing the credit he had allowed them and that he was depressed.

I can still see the look of concern on Dr. Allen's face as he walked toward me. He was an ex-Marine and was used to hearing bad news. I told him, through my tears, what had happened.

Dr. Allen said, "Dave, I am so sorry. You need to go home and take care of your family. Take as much time as you need."

I did. I helped with the funeral arrangements and tried to support Mom, who was a sweet, stoic little woman. But it was not an easy time. A day after the funeral, I went into the shed in the backyard where Dad had taken his life. On the floor, I saw the 12-gauge shotgun and the small ball-peen hammer he had used to push the trigger.

One of the hardest things I have ever had to do was go in that shed where Dad stored a little bit of everything, from lumber to lawnmowers, and clean up his blood and brains that had splattered over everything.

Late the night before Dad took his life and after Mom had gone to bed, he had written a short note to her and put an insurance policy worth approximately $30,000, listing her as the beneficiary, on the dining room table. In his depression, he couldn't think straight. His business was failing, and he was in debt to the First National Bank for about $40,000, primarily because his customers were taking advantage of his generosity and not paying their bills for the groceries they bought on credit.

But despite being deeply in debt — $40,000 was a lot of money back in 1974 — his situation was not as dire as he thought it to be. Dad owned our home and our cabin on the Cowpasture River, so he could have erased his debt by selling our cabin, which was in a very desirable location on one of the most beautiful rivers in Virginia. But he couldn't bring himself to do that. He loved that cabin as much as life itself. He knew he couldn't retire; he didn't have any retirement plan. His plan had always been to work until he died. That's what you do when you own a small business that is your only source of income.

I never had any bitterness about Dad's suicide. I knew that when a person's mood gets so low, suicide may seem like an easy way out. I vaguely understood depression and bipolar disorder. I also came to understand that bipolar disorder runs in my dad's side of the family. He had four brothers — one committed suicide when he was a young man and the other three, like Dad, were functioning alcoholics. I believe that they used alcohol to treat their depression, just like Dad did. Dad's three living brothers were all successful in their careers, and they all had long marriages to the same women. And although I know there must have been many tough times in those marriages, none of the three let alcohol destroy them.

My Mom had also stayed strong. She had always been shy and rather introverted — traits I inherited from her — but she would stand up for what she thought was right. To me, Mom was the sweetest little woman, and I loved her so much. She was also so beautiful that she had been named "best looking" in her high school senior class superlatives. Though she did not approve of Dad's drinking, she was pretty stoic about it and never caused any scenes when that topic occasionally came up, at least not in front of us children.

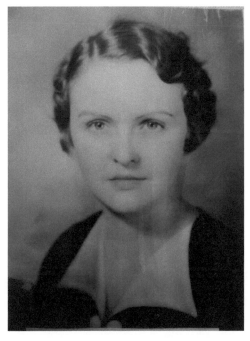

Mom, just before she married my dad in 1935

MOM'S HEALTH, HOWEVER, HAD never been good. Yet even with her rheumatic heart and three children, she always had a hot meal for the family, three times a day, every single day. She ordered our groceries from The Food Center, did the laundry and house cleaning for all of us with only occasional help from a caregiver after her stroke. Even with all that to do, Mom often helped out at Dad's store, working as one of his clerks on busy Saturdays.

She was even-tempered and seldom gave us kids a spanking, or even a severe scolding. I personally don't think I ever got a spanking, although I am sure I deserved more than one. She was always extremely supportive and encouraging. I couldn't have asked for more in a Mom.

When my mother was 49, she had a serious stroke which left her left side paralyzed for about six months. Shortly after her stroke, she had open-heart surgery at the University of Virginia medical hospital in Charlottesville to replace a faulty valve. Her surgery was performed by a Dr. Julian Beckwith, the father of a good friend who was a high school classmate of mine. Mom's heart had such an unusual rhythm from her rheumatic fever that, before her operation, Dr. Beckwith had all the young interns come into her room and listen to it. Mom would recover from the stroke and the surgery despite her rheumatic heart disease.

My mother was honest to a fault. She would not even tell a "little white lie." I inherited this trait from her, but possibly not to the same degree as her. Heck, being a fisherman, I am expected to exaggerate a little bit. You may have heard the old question, "Are all fishermen liars, or do only liars fish?" There is probably a little truth in both of those propositions, especially the first one.

My honesty, and lack of tact, occasionally got me in trouble. I remember having a conversation with Mom and Dad as we were finishing our evening meal. I was in college at the time and home for the weekend. I was standing beside Dad with my hand on his shoulder and said, "I am so lucky to have a hard-working father and an honest mother." But as soon as I said it, I knew it didn't come out right. Dad looked up at me and, with a smile, said, "Are you saying I'm not honest?"

I was trying to pay both of them a compliment, letting them know that I appreciated their good traits. I'm just glad Dad was a good sport about it. It was just one of many experiences that taught me to think before I opened my mouth.

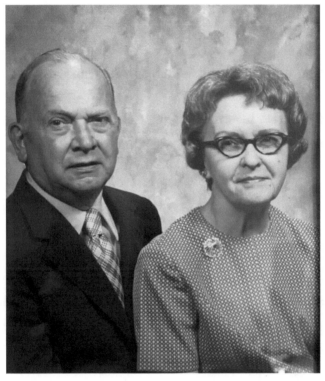

My hardworking dad and my honest mom in 1970

IN HIGH SCHOOL, I bonded with Dad more than my brother Eddy did. Dad and Eddy loved each other, but they had a difficult time bonding. Eddy's mental makeup was too similar to Dad's for them to hit it off together. We didn't know it at that time, but Eddy was later diagnosed with bipolar disorder. When his mood was stable, he was as sweet and nice a person as could be. Eddy was extremely popular in high school, good looking, president of his senior class and a good athlete — a linebacker on the football team and right fielder on the baseball team.

But Eddy's manic behavior began to express itself in high school. I remember watching a football practice one day when Eddy must have been in a manic state. The offensive line couldn't keep him out of their backfield. He just kept bursting through on every snap of the ball, getting into the backfield, like a wild man. Finally, the coach said, "Van Lear, go take a shower."

While Dad had begun taking me fishing when I was about 11 or 12, Eddy never liked to fish with Dad like I did. We did have a sort of "hunting tradition" that we all shared. Even though I was much more interested in fishing than hunting, Eddy and I would hunt squirrels with my dad on Thanksgiving. Since Dad knew about everyone in the county and was good friends with most of them, we would hunt on the properties of landowners who had given him permission. We used 22-caliber Winchester rifles. His was a pump action model 61, I believe, and mine was a bolt action model 69. Eddy had a lever-action 22 rifle that he used when he went with us. We often killed a few squirrels, and Mom would make squirrel stew for supper when we got home.

Right after his high school graduation, Eddy joined the Marines and was sent off to Parris Island, South Carolina, for boot camp. He was deeply in love with a girl from a neighboring high school at the time. After about 10 weeks at Parris Island, near the end of boot camp, Eddy received a "Dear John" letter from her. Shortly thereafter he had what was called a "nervous breakdown." He was honorably discharged and came back home.

After coming home, Eddy lived in an upstairs bedroom in our family's house with the shades pulled and stayed to himself as much as possible for months, as I recall. He was so ashamed and depressed.

Finally, a neighbor who lived across the street told Mom and Dad about Bob Jones University, a fundamentalist Christian university in Greenville, South Carolina, thinking that the school's strict religious views were just what Eddy needed to get him back on track. Eddy gave it a try but didn't last long there — less than one semester. Eddy just didn't "buy the goods" that Bob Jones was selling and within a few months was back home with Mom and Dad.

Early the following spring, several of Eddy's high school friends were taking a trip to the west coast and invited him to go with them. When they reached Wyoming, they were running short of money. A couple of them, including Eddy, were dropped off at Yellowstone National Park in hopes that they could get summer jobs there; they did. Yellowstone National Park turned out to be one of the best things that ever happened to Eddy.

The next summer, he went back to Yellowstone when he was offered the job of Superintendent of Services at Old Faithful Camper Cabins, which meant he was the boss of about 12 bellhops. Eddy loved Yellowstone and urged me to apply for a summer job when I graduated from high school the next year. He said, "It will change your life." And he was definitely right.

The following fall, Eddy enrolled at Bridgewater College in Bridgewater, Virginia. He was a member of the football team and had the distinction during his junior year of rooming with the college's first Black student. Eddy was a leader, just like Dad, doing the right thing, even if it was unpopular in segregationist Virginia in the early 1960s.

Eddy graduated from Bridgewater with a major in philosophy and a minor in history. He came back home to Clifton Forge and was hired by the high school to teach history. There, he met his wife, Lillian, who was a teacher there also. After their two children, Edward and Mark, were born, Eddy and Lil enrolled in James Madison University to pursue master's degrees.

But teaching high school, earning a master's degree (he was revising the final draft of his thesis) and being a husband and father to two young boys at the same time, took too much of a toll on Eddy's fragile bipolar mind. He had another "nervous breakdown" and was admitted to Western State Psychiatric Hospital in Staunton, Virginia.

In 1974, Eddy tried to go back to teaching, but he was on so much medication that he couldn't do it. The medication made him zombie-like, and he left school abruptly one morning early in the school year and went home. When the principal told Lillian that Eddy had just walked out of his classroom, she left school and went home to check on him. There, she found Eddy was in a darkened upstairs bedroom with his rifle in his hands.

He said, "Lil, I just can't do it anymore. My life is over."

Lil walked calmly over to him, took the gun from his hands and told him that there was help for him. He didn't resist. Shortly afterward, Lil and I took Eddy to St. Albans Mental Hospital in Radford, Virginia, where he was given 12 electrical shock treatments, evidently the standard treatment at the time for people coming off nervous breakdowns and who were considered suicidal.

Those treatments didn't help Eddy much. He tried to commit suicide once at St. Albans, but the second-floor window he tried to smash himself through didn't collapse; it just gave him a bloody head.

A few years later, Eddy finally got a big break. Doctors put him on lithium, a medicine that had been shown to be effective in calming moods. The medicine was highly effective in treating Eddy and allowed him to function, at least without suicidal thoughts, for 25 years or more, but eventually it destroyed his kidney function.

Eddy refused to go on dialysis. Life had been too tough on him, and he had had enough. In 2010, Eddy died from kidney failure. Everyone in our family understood his struggles. Eddy's wife, Lil, an angel to the end, took care of him for decades as he battled his bipolar condition.

My sister Kitty who is four years younger than me was an excellent student and was valedictorian of her high school graduating class. Kitty went to Mary Washington College (now the University of Mary Washington) in Fredericksburg, Virginia, and majored in German with the goal of becoming a German teacher. She went on to receive a master's degree in German from the University of Virginia.

After graduating with her M.F.A., Kitty was a very successful German teacher in the Virginia Beach school system for decades. She was highly rated by her students and took many of her classes on summer field trips to Germany.

Chapter 3

Finding My First Love — Smallmouth Bass

WHILE IT MAY INTERRUPT the chronology of my story, I cannot really move forward in my narrative without talking about my first true love: fishing.

The first major turning point in my life occurred in 1952 when my dad bought a two-acre lot about seven miles from our home in Clifton Forge, on the Cowpasture River, still one of the most beautiful and unspoiled rivers in Virginia. Dad and a friend named Bob Brown worked in the evenings after their regular jobs to help contractors build a summer cabin for us on the river. Dad was very handy and could do just about anything needed to help build our cabin.

When Dad finished our cabin, he bought a small wooden jon boat that I would paddle across the river and fish for smallmouth bass, bluegills and redbreast. In those first years on the river, I fished with live bait, then with artificial spinning lures and later with flies. Each form of fishing enhanced my enjoyment and gave me a way to cope with the occasional sad times that I would experience.

The family cabin

THE COWPASTURE RIVER THAT ran beside our cabin is where I caught my first large smallmouth bass and became a serious fisherman when I was just 12 years old, an event that set the stage for a lifelong addiction and a hobby that has never left me.

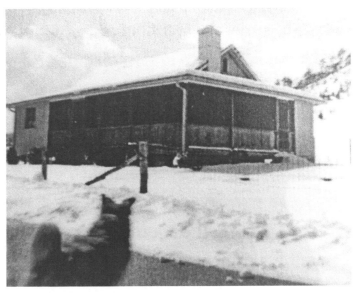

Sparky at our cabin on the Cowpasture River

OUR FAMILY LIVED IN the cabin from the time high school was out in early June until well into the fall, when we would move back into town. The cabin had three bedrooms, a living room, a kitchen, bathroom and a large wrap-around, screened-in porch. We all loved both the cabin and the river so much that the place helped the family bond.

My dad and I loved to fish for smallmouth bass and other species in the Cowpasture River and Craig's Creek, cool, clear-water streams close to Clifton Forge. Dad traditionally closed his store on Wednesday afternoons giving us time to fish sections of the rivers that flowed through private property owned by local doctors and farmers he knew, several of whom did business with Dad at his grocery store.

When we wanted to go fishing, Dad and I would load the wooden jon boat in the back of his delivery truck and head out to one of the rivers we normally fished. When we got home late in the evening, Mom would fry up the fish we caught, usually a mixture of smallmouth bass, bluegills and redbreasts, with an occasional pickerel or channel catfish, and we would talk about our afternoon as we ate a delicious supper. Fishing gave Dad and me a way to bond, and when we built the cabin, fishing was just off our front porch. I remember well my first big catch. I was 12 years old and fishing out of Dad's jon boat in front of our cabin. Fishing was pretty good, and I had caught a few small bass and a couple of bluegills on the spring lizards I was using for bait. In those early years, Dad and I used live bait like spring lizards, cat minnows and hellgrammites.

I cast again and had a nibble on my lizard. I jerked and had a fish on for a second — then bam, something much bigger slammed that little fish. I struck again and was fast to a big smallmouth bass that had tried to eat the panfish that had nibbled my lizard and got hooked itself. The big fish immediately made a run, making the drag on my Johnson Century sing for a few seconds. I had never had a fish do that! The big fish came to the surface and jumped about ten feet from the boat, scaring the hell out of me!

Since I had never caught a big fish before, I wasn't exactly sure how to get it in the boat. So, I did exactly what you should *not* do. Instead of grabbing the bass by its lower jaw when it got close to the boat, I tried to lift the fish out of the water with my fiberglass rod, hoping to swing it into the boat. While it was swinging, the fish jerked off the hook. Thankfully, it landed in the bottom of the boat, and I was on it in a flash.

Suppose that bass, instead of landing in the boat had landed in the river and escaped? Would I have become the avid angler that I became? I don't know. I just know that I had caught a three-pound smallmouth bass, a very nice bass for the Cowpasture River, and the seeds of my addiction to fishing — with all its mental and physical benefits — had been sown.

By the time I was a junior in high school, I was using artificial lures as much as live bait, but my dad stuck with live bait. When spincast reels, like the Johnson Century and Zebco 33, came into style in the 1950s, they just added to my enjoyment of fishing.

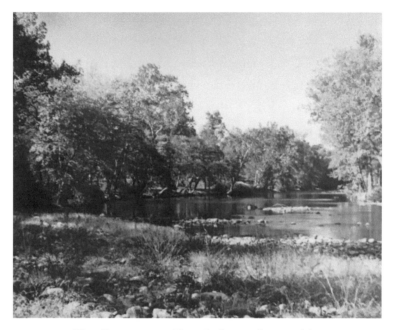

The Cowpasture River in front of our cabin

I USED DAD'S JON boat to fish the deeper, more "fishy looking," far side of the river in front of our cabin. Sometimes I would pull the boat upstream through the rapids to the next eddy, where I caught my largest smallmouth when I was in my early 20s. Although I caught many fish on artificial lures, I caught most of my large smallmouth bass, anything over two pounds, on cat minnows, our favorite bait for big smallmouth bass. My largest weighed 4¼ pounds.

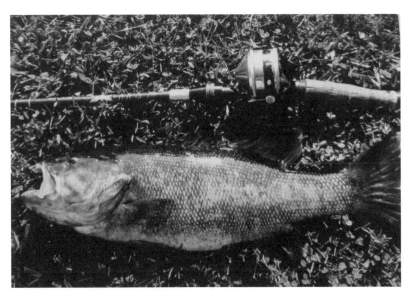

My largest smallmouth bass, a 4¼ pounder from the
Cowpasture River

MY DAD AND I fished the Cowpasture River and Craig's Creek almost
exclusively. However, on a few occasions, my uncle Earl took me fishing on the Calfpasture River, a smaller version of the Cowpasture.

I sometimes fished for stocked trout in small, swift, rocky creeks
near my hometown, and I occasionally fished the headwaters of these
trout streams for native brook trout, trout too small to satisfy most
fishermen. In high school, my favorite baits for trout were night-
crawlers and minnows. I had not yet been hooked on fly fishing.

My whole family loved the cabin that Dad had provided for us,
but for me, as an "outdoorsy" type, there couldn't have been a better
place to grow up. As a teenager, I would swim and fish in the river
practically every day during the summer and into the fall until cold
weather would drive us back to Clifton Forge. The cabin and the river beside it helped shape the person I would become in both my ca-

reer and my lifelong love of fishing. Fishing, particularly fly fishing, would return again and again in my life story.

Fishing with a little hunting on the side

IN HIGH SCHOOL, I was not much of a big game hunter. I only went deer hunting a few times and was lucky just once while hunting on land owned by the grandfather of my best friend, Richard Deeds. Sitting mid-slope on an oak-dominated hillside, I caught a glimpse out of the corner of my eye of a buck sneaking up the ridgeline on the next hill over. He was about 80 yards away.

I slowly twisted around and raised my rifle, a .30-06 I had borrowed from Richard and later bought from him. The buck must have seen me move, because it stopped and looked my way. Though I had fired Richard's gun only a few times, I squeezed off a shot, aiming for a spot just behind the buck's shoulder.

The buck, an eight-pointer with a heavy rack, immediately went down. I had hustled over to put my tag on him, when a small group of older hunters came out of nowhere it seemed to me and started acting like my deer was their deer. Thankfully, Richard's dad showed up and quickly put a stop to that nonsense. And my proud Dad had the buck's head mounted for me.

Chapter 4

The Glory of Yellowstone

ALWAYS, FOR ME, MY heart was in the fishing. I have my brother Eddy to thank for introducing me to some of the wildest and most beautiful waters in the world. Eddy urged me to go to Yellowstone National Park and work, telling me that the experience would change my life. He was correct, and that decision to go to Yellowstone became another turning point in my life.

When I graduated from high school in 1958, my best friend Richard Deeds and I went to Yellowstone National Park for summer jobs. We cleaned the tourist cabins at Old Faithful, one of the busiest tourist destinations in the park. Richard and I lived in barracks owned by the Yellowstone Park Company for park employees. There was no glamour in the jobs, but what a place to fuel an addiction to fishing.

Richard and I had fished for trout in the small creeks around our hometown in Virginia, but we had never experienced trout fishing like we would find in Yellowstone. It seemed like our lucky summer, beginning with a conversation with an old man who worked in the fishing department of Hamilton Stores, a concessionaire in the park, who saved our summer of fishing. Richard and I had fished for a couple of weeks with our fly rods trying to catch trout on the fly-fishing-only Firehole River, to no avail. Finally, we asked the old man behind the counter if he knew of a stream we could fish with our spinning rods. He told us about a stream he once fished called Iron Creek.

Our barracks were only a 15-minute hike through the woods from Iron Creek. After cleaning our allotted cabins, which we generally accomplished by about three o'clock in the afternoon, we would grab our fishing rods and walk the mile through the woods behind our barracks to this beautiful meadow stream that flowed through Black Sand Basin. It was loaded with wild brown and rainbow trout and, in its upper reaches, even had eastern brook trout. Richard and I fished this stream as often as two or three times a week.

We seemed to be the only ones fishing Iron Creek that summer, and we caught loads of trout, including a four-pound brown trout that Richard caught — our largest catch of the summer.

What more could a fisherman have hoped for? We had a tranquil meadow stream full of wild trout that seemed to be all ours and plenty of time to fish.

Though Richard could not go back to the park after that first summer, I continued to work as a bellhop for four more summers, working one summer at Old Faithful Inn and three at Canyon Village, all while I pursued my Bachelor of Science and Master of Science in forestry at Virginia Tech.

The beauty and uniqueness of Yellowstone, as well as the fishing and the gathering of old friends from all over the country, year after year, kept drawing me back to the park. In fact, I'd say Yellowstone

National Park and fly fishing have become completely intertwined in my addiction, and during my 80-plus years of life, I have returned to Yellowstone 30 to 40 times.

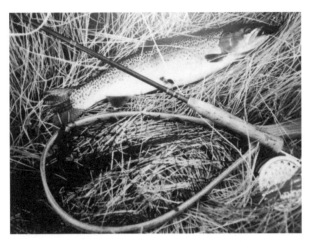

Rainbow trout from Yellowstone's Madison River

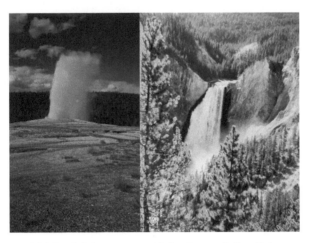

Old Faithful geyser and the lower falls of the
Yellowstone River

Chapter 5

The Lure of Fly Fishing

DURING THOSE SUMMERS WORKING in the park, I gradually switched from spin fishing to fly fishing, and my addiction to the sport became stronger. I loved everything about fly fishing, from the longer rods to the relatively tiny flies on the end of my leader, to the gorgeous environments of trout streams, to the surreal beauty of the trout themselves. The almost hypnotic movement of the heavy fly line as it is cast back and forth, lengthening the cast to the distance needed, simply contributed to my addiction.

I have one vivid recollection of the occasion which triggered my switching from spin fishing to fly fishing. In 1959, my second summer working in Yellowstone, I was attempting to fly fish (I use the term loosely, because I was a novice to be sure) a stretch of the Firehole River just upstream from Biscuit Basin. I noticed an older gentleman fly fishing in the riffle-run ahead of me. As I watched him making short casts directly upstream of his position, he caught and released two nice trout in just a few minutes.

Standing there in awe, I suddenly heard and saw a splashy rise off in a slough to my right, on the other side of the river. As I intently gazed at the riseform, I noticed a couple of dragonflies darting about above the quiet surface of the water. "Darn," I thought. "They are jumping after those dragonflies!"

I knew what dragonflies were from my summers growing up on the Cowpasture River but I didn't have anything in my meager fly box to represent them, so I picked out the biggest, bushiest fly I had and knotted it onto my tippet.

As quietly as I possibly could, I waded across the Firehole until I was close enough for even me to make a cast to where I had seen the rise. Glory be! I made a good cast that landed the fly two feet above the spot where the fish rose. And sure enough a nice trout rose and slurped the big fly into its mouth. I struck and was fast to a big brown trout.

After a spirited fight, I was able to net the fish and take it to the bank. Wow! It was 18 inches long at least, by far the biggest trout I had caught in my first two summers working in Yellowstone, and I had caught it on a fly. From that point on I was hooked on fly fishing.

I quickly took my prize catch upstream to show it to the old man who was still fishing the same riffle-run where I had first seen him. He waded over to the bank to see my fish. He was very friendly and complimented me on a fine catch.

Then he did something that I didn't expect. He took my fish, which was still alive and kicking, and snapped its neck and gave it back to me. He said, "Son, we don't want our treasures to suffer when we keep them, do we?"

The old man's sentiments and actions made a deep impression on me, and as I think back, probably were the beginning of my becoming a "catch and release" fly fishing advocate.

As we walked back to the parking lot at Biscuit Basin, the old man told me that he had been fishing the waters of Yellowstone for decades and considered them to be the best trout streams in the United States. I wish I had gotten the old man's name because I have often wondered if he might not have been one of the angling editors of a popular outdoor magazine of the 1950s, perhaps Joe Brooks, Ray Bergman, or Ted Trueblood, writers that I later learned spent much time in Yellowstone. Probably not, but I like to think he might have been.

While Yellowstone is known to most people for its wildlife, waterfalls and thermal features, as well as its cultural features, like Old Faithful Inn and Canyon Village, it is known to fishermen, especially fly fisherman, for its outstanding trout fishing. The park is home to many famous trout streams, such as the Madison, Yellowstone, Firehole, Gibbon and Lamar rivers and I have fished them all many times in my 60-plus years of visiting the park.

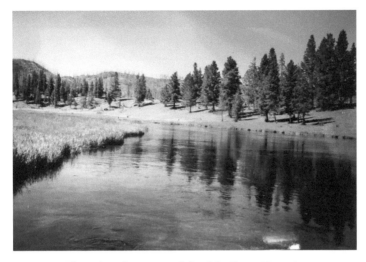

The placid waters of the Madison River in
Yellowstone National Park

THE PARK ALSO HAS dozens, if not hundreds, of small, trout-filled streams, such as Iron, Grayling and DeLacy creeks, to name just a few of those I've fished.

Seeing the park's wildlife, especially elk and bison, is often an added bonus when fishing these streams. However, Yellowstone is wilderness, and I was always a little apprehensive when I fished alone on park streams, especially if I was some distance away from the road. Because of my uneasiness when fishing alone in bear country, I kept up a rather loud conservation with my imaginary fishing buddy, "Fred," using two voice tones, to let any bears that might be in the neighborhood think that I wasn't alone.

Just once did that strategy fail me.

Late in the summer of 1961, two of my bellhop friends and I drove from our jobs in Canyon Village to Iron Creek for an afternoon of fishing. We parked in the parking lot for Black Sand Basin and began putting on our gear. My friends had their spinning gear ready to go before I could thread my fly line through all the guides on my 8½-foot fly rod and put on my waders.

Finally, I was rigged up and ready to go, but by that time my buddies had already started fishing downstream from the geyser basin. I didn't want to fish behind them, thinking that they would have spooked the trout, making them more difficult for me to catch, so I hiked upstream of the basin and began fishing.

I had fished upstream for about a half mile, catching a few small trout, but was beginning to feel a little anxious about my situation, knowing that grizzlies had been reported in the area of the nearby Firehole River, and I was all alone. My buddies by now were probably a mile below Black Sand Basin.

When I had started fishing upstream a couple hours earlier, there had been a few tourists walking the boardwalk at Morning Glory pool, one of the most famous thermal features in Black Sand Basin, but I was far away from that spot now.

The forest and grassy meadow along Iron Creek, soggy and ripe with mosquitos even though it was late in the summer, suddenly seemed unnaturally quiet. Still talking rather loudly to "Fred," I climbed out of the stream and crept along the west bank, sneaking up on the next fishy looking run. I began to feel I wasn't alone on the stream. It was just too quiet. I would soon see the reason why.

As I rounded a bend in the stream, there — no more than 30 yards away — stood a mother grizzly and her two half-grown cubs, staring right at me, probably wondering, "Who the hell is he talking to?" The grizzlies were on the same side of the creek as me, so close that I could have cast my fly to them. I knew that with just a few bounds they could be on me and have me for lunch. I had read enough stories about grizzly attacks and maulings that I knew running into a mother grizzly with two cubs was extremely dangerous.

No, these were not black bears. I was very familiar with black bears, having helped chase dozens of them away from the garbage cans they raided when I worked at Old Faithful camper cabins and the lodge at Canyon Village. There was no doubt in my mind that these were grizzly bears.

They had the "dished-in" faces, the pronounced hump on their backs, and the grizzled brown fur — all distinctive characteristics of grizzlies. Grizzlies, I knew, were a much more formidable bear than the black bear, and these grizzlies weren't moving away.

But what should I do? The mother bear could be on me in seconds and maul me into pieces. I knew I couldn't outrun them. Grizzlies can outrun the fastest human sprinters, and I certainly wasn't one of those, particularly not while wearing waders. And I did not want to trigger a predator-prey response in those bears by running. After all, I would be the prey!

The grizzlies were still looking at me as I began slowly to back away. For some reason, I began making a low moaning sound, thinking — I don't know why — the sound might make the bears sense I wasn't afraid. And I wasn't afraid — I was *terrified*! I thought my heart would pound out of my chest.

I had backed away a few yards when I stumbled and fell over a dead lodgepole pine tree, one of millions, if not billions, of such trees lying on the forest floor in the park. When I fell, I dropped my fly rod and my pipe slipped out of my mouth. As I cautiously got to my feet, the mother bear jerked her head, and her cubs immediately turned and ran back behind her into the dense woods.

Now it was just mama bear and me staring at each other from a distance of perhaps 35 yards. Looking behind me, I saw two pine trees growing about three feet apart. I moved very slowly toward them, keeping a wary eye on the bear all the time. When I reached the two, six- to seven-inch-diameter trees, I placed myself between them and, with the help of a major adrenaline rush, spread-eagled my way up to the lowest live branches, which were about 12 to 15 feet above the ground. Then I climbed over to the largest of the two trees and climbed farther up, until I was about 20 feet off the ground.

Now I was feeling a little safer.

In 1961, common knowledge said that adult grizzlies do not climb trees — at least that is what I thought the common knowledge said. Today a quick internet search will tell you that adult grizzlies can indeed climb trees. However, back in the 1960s, the consensus of the many stories I had read was to avoid a grizzly attack by climbing a tree with no low branches, and this was no time to test the "grizzlies can climb/can't climb" hypothesis.

While I was climbing up those two trees, the mother grizzly started walking slowly toward me. She came within about 20 feet of my tree, and I remember looking down on her and seeing the brownish-silver hair on her back standing straight up, "like a mad dog's," I remember thinking. Her eyes looked like black obsidian.

She stood there for a few seconds, looking up at me, and then turned and headed back into the woods where the cubs had run. I decided to stay up in the tree a while longer and, it's a good thing I did. About 10 minutes later, the bear came back to where I had originally seen her with the cubs. She didn't seem to want to leave that spot. I later thought that maybe the bears had been eating an elk calf that they had killed, and that was why they didn't run into the woods when "Fred" and I were approaching, talking loudly to each other. Normally, bears will move away if they hear people approaching, unless they are guarding food.

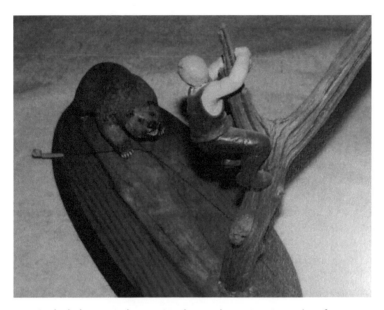

A slightly over-dramatized wood carving I made of me climbing a tree to escape a charging grizzly who stomped on and broke my fly rod

FINALLY, MAMA BEAR LEFT. I stayed up that pine tree for about 45 minutes more, afraid to climb down. Finally, not seeing any sign of her, I climbed down to the lowest dead limb, dropped to the ground, grabbed my fishing rod (I didn't take the time to look for my pipe), hopped across Iron Creek in two or three bounds, ran until breathless, then walked very rapidly across a long grassy meadow back to Black Sand Basin where I was safe at last and with a memory that I thought would last a lifetime. And it has.

Incidentally, I believe that mother grizzly and her two cubs were killed later that summer by National Park Service rangers. There were numerous bear-fishermen incidents reported in 1961 near the Firehole River, and they had escalated as the summer progressed until it became necessary for the National Park Service to remove, or kill, the bears.

Two summers later, in 1963, the last summer I worked in the park, I visited the Canyon Village visitor center. There, I saw a mother grizzly with two cubs that had been mounted in a pose that looked eerily similar to the bears I saw on Iron Creek. Much later, in 2008, while my wife Carolyn and I were visiting the park, a ranger at the Fishing Bridge Visitor Center, where a mounted mother grizzly and two half-grown cubs were being displayed, told me that those bears were killed in 1961, the same year I was treed. I would bet they were "my" bears.

Working in Yellowstone those five summers, among the forests, rivers and waterfalls, wildlife, geysers and spectacular scenery, was a major turning point in my life as it reinforced my leaning toward a career in a natural resources field. I chose to major in forest management at Virginia Tech.

Chapter 6

Education at the Next Level

I WAS AN AVERAGE student in high school. With minimal effort I was able to make B's and C's, with occasional A's — satisfactory grades, at least satisfactory to me. There was no tradition in my family of putting great emphasis on education. I had no plans of going to college, in fact, I hadn't even thought about it.

My dad had gone to the University of Richmond for two years but had dropped out for financial reasons during the Great Depression of the 1930s. And although his living brothers had successful careers, he was the only male in his family to have any college experience.

So, I just kind of "slid" through high school, not putting much effort into academic achievement. I was well liked and served as a class officer. And while I wanted to do well in my classes, I evidently did not want it enough to study hard. I did not see the need to make straight A's.

My major effort in high school was to make the basketball team. When I was 12 years old and entering the 8th grade at Clifton Forge

High School, I foolishly went out for the JV football team. I was small for my age and only weighed about 110 pounds, but because my brother was a 200-pound linebacker on the varsity football team, I thought I could play as well. I made the team — almost everybody did — but it was obvious I was too small to be a football player. I was pretty tough for my size, but in football, size does make a difference.

Besides, I loved basketball much more than I did football. I was on the junior varsity basketball team in my freshman and sophomore years, but finally made the varsity team in my junior and senior years. In my senior year, I was a starting guard on the team — not a big scorer to be sure but a pretty good ball handler and assist man. We had a very good team and won the regular season championship of District 5 with a 15-5 record, but eventually lost out in the district tournament.

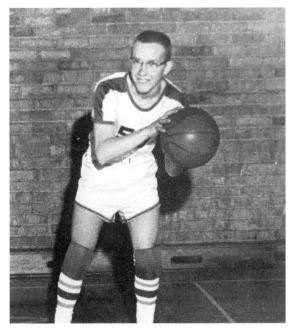

I played guard on our Clifton Forge High School
basketball team

I WAS POPULAR AND served as president of the student council my
senior year, but I certainly was not a ladies' man in high school, perhaps because I was a small guy and just naturally bashful. Besides
being shy around girls, I didn't have much money for dating, and I
didn't have a nice car to impress the girls, like some of my friends. I
had occasional dates, like for major dances, but never had a steady
girl in high school, even though I had secret crushes on a couple of
pretty girls.

My family lived on a street that connected the high school to
downtown Clifton Forge, and I can remember many times sitting in
the front room of our house after school, watching through the cur-
tains as boys and girls walked by on their way to Farrar's Drug Store

where they could buy a soda and socialize. Sadly, I was just too shy and didn't have the money to join in the fun.

So, while I might not have been the happiest kid in high school, I still considered myself relatively lucky. I was a good athlete, although too small to be a star, an average student and had a loving family, a wonderful cabin on a beautiful river, a great dog and a hobby that made me happy and helped me through tough times in my life.

But what was I going to do with the rest of my life after high school?

In 1958, I was a senior in high school and besides being president of the student council, was president of our Presbyterian Church youth group. One evening, when that group was meeting at the home of our minister, Dr. Phillip Roberts, he casually asked me what I was going to do next year. I told him I had not given it much thought but would probably look for a job in town, although there weren't many of those around. Dr. Roberts told me I would need a college education to be competitive and productive in society, and he thought I should consider college.

Dr. Roberts was a respected preacher with an excellent reputation in the state. He had strong ties to a Presbyterian liberal arts college named Hampden-Sydney, which I discovered was a highly rated all-male college and one of the oldest colleges in the country.

Dr. Roberts told me he might be able to get me into Hampden-Sydney, despite my average grades. I learned that the college had a strong academic reputation that went back nearly 200 years, to 1775. Patrick Henry and James Madison had been on Hampden-Sydney's first board of trustees — not too shabby.

I was accepted, thanks to Dr. Roberts' influence, and entered the freshman class in the fall of 1958. Going to Hampden-Sydney College was one of the most important turning points in my life. Who knows what I would have become if I had not gone to college?

At Hampden-Sydney I was finally motivated to do my best academically, something I had never done. First, I wanted to redeem my parents' faith in me. Although I did get several small scholarships at Hampden-Sydney based on need, not my high school academic performance for sure, my parents paid my way through undergraduate school, and they encouraged me every day.

While I was able to get student loans to help pay my tuition and other expenses later at Virginia Tech, Dad had to borrow from the First National Bank to pay for my time at Hampden-Sydney, something he never complained about. He was proud of me for doing something he hadn't been able to do when he was forced to leave the University of Richmond after just two years.

My second motivation to do well at Hampden-Sydney was to live up to the trust that Dr. Roberts had in me. He must have seen something in me that I hadn't seen in myself. And because Dr. Roberts and my parents had faith in me, I was determined to do well academically at Hampden-Sydney or die trying. Fear of failure was becoming a life-long motivating factor that helped me in college and throughout my career. Being afraid to fail helped me succeed, and success made me feel good about myself.

I also thought my parents needed some good news. Eddy, my big brother, was holed up in an upstairs bedroom with the shades drawn, after leaving the Marines. He was trying to deal with his depression and shame. Though I was still in high school when Eddy came home from the Marines and a little too young to understand the gravity of his situation, I could see that it was taking a toll on Mom and Dad.

I thought that perhaps I could deliver that news by doing well in college.

For all those motivations, I really buckled down and studied hard, for the first time in my life, when I enrolled in Hampden-Sydney. Many of the students at Hampden-Sydney were sons of lawyers and doctors, came from wealthy homes and had excellent academic backgrounds. They were stiff competitors academically, but I had always been a competitive person, at least athletically, and here, I found that if I studied hard I could keep up with them academically. Indeed, I found that I could actually do better than most of them, not because I was smarter but because I studied harder.

Most of the students at Hampden-Sydney were accustomed to having it relatively easy, at least financially, compared to me. Nearly all of them joined expensive fraternities and had cars. I didn't have the time or money to join one of the social fraternities and certainly didn't own a car. When I wanted to go home on a weekend, I would have to hitch a ride with one of my friends from Clifton Forge or hitchhike. I didn't have any interest in joining a fraternity — frankly, I thought they were kind of silly.

Hampden-Sydney, although a college with a very good academic standing, was a big party school, and I wasn't there to party. I was there to learn and excel. Money was tight for me and in my sophomore year, I delivered newspapers on campus just to earn a little spending money.

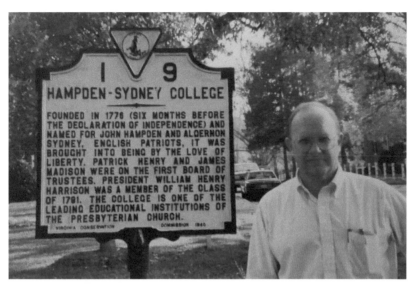

All freshmen were required to memorize the words on this plaque when they arrived on campus. This photo was taken when I revisited the campus about 20 years ago.

WHILE AT HAMPDEN-SYDNEY I enjoyed playing intramural softball and basketball. And although most of my memories of playing sports there are pleasant, my time in sports did include a few unpleasant memories. The first happened after a softball game when I decided to take a shortcut alone through the woods back to my dorm. It was during preparations for the 1960 summer Olympics, and I had enjoyed watching them on TV as often as I could, especially the sprinting events.

I was a pretty fast runner and on this particular day I was sprinting through the woods, dreaming I was an Olympic sprinter. In my path ahead I saw a stack of cross ties about three-feet high. I suddenly became a hurdler as well as a sprinter and, as I started to hurdle over the cross ties as fast as I could go, I saw a strand of barbed wire suddenly appear above the cross ties. As my neck collided with the fence, I was thrown violently to the ground.

Dazed and bleeding from the neck, I knew there was no one around to help me. Gradually, after a few minutes, I was able to gather my senses, get to my feet and find my way back to the dorm. Luckily, the barbed wire did not cut my jugular vein or carotid artery. It just left a rather nasty two-inch scar on the right side of my neck which I carry to this day.

Another memorable intramural moment happened during a basketball game. During the game, I accidently caught an elbow that shattered my glasses into my left eye. One of my teammates (I have unforgivably forgotten his name, though I can remember what he looked like) took me immediately to the campus infirmary. There, the college doctor, a grand old man, probably in his late 70s, tried without success to remove glass splinters from my eye. He just couldn't see well enough to do the job.

Thankfully, my teammate had much better eyesight and was able to remove two or three glass splinters from my eye. Luckily, I suffered no lasting damage to my eye from the accident.

My academic career did not afford the same dangers. And through hard work, I excelled academically at Hampden-Sydney, majoring in liberal arts with an emphasis on Latin. Latin, you say! Yes, I had taken two years of the language in high school and took two more years at Hampden-Sydney and felt comfortable with the subject. I did well in Latin and actually in all my classes at Hampden-Sydney, ranking fourth in my class of about 150 at the end of my sophomore year.

I certainly didn't realize it at the time, but the two years I spent at Hampden-Sydney College in a liberal arts curriculum really played a major role in shaping my life. I found that I could excel academically, something I had never known in high school. Taking courses in history, chemistry, algebra, philosophy, ethics, English composition and literature, French and Latin, as well as courses in the Old and New Testament, gave me a much broader perspective on life and laid the groundwork for my career in an applied natural science such as forestry.

I don't necessarily attribute my academic success to being extremely intelligent; I attribute it more to studying hard, being afraid of failure and always doing my best. By this time in my life, I was beginning to think that being mildly bipolar had something to do with my success, too. I often sought out the successes of famous people such as Winston Churchill, Henry Ford, Ernest Hemingway and others, who did amazing things even though diagnosed with bipolar disorder, or manic depression as it was called back then. To me, these people were role models of how it is possible to succeed despite having mental illness.

I knew that even with his bipolar disorder my dad had held his own against overwhelming odds for decades — going on to lead in his school, church and community. And I hoped I could do the same.

After a couple years at Hampden-Sydney, I knew I wasn't cut out to be a Latin scholar or Latin teacher. My interest was in the outdoors, an interest enhanced by working summers in Yellowstone National Park, where the beauty of nature — forests, streams, wildlife, geysers and hot springs — all worked their magic on me.

In 1960 I came to the next major turning point in my life. I decided, at the end of my sophomore year, to transfer from Hampden-Sydney to Virginia Tech to major in forest management.

Chapter 7

Turning Toward My Career

TRANSFERRING TO VIRGINIA TECH was a great move for me, and I loved most of my courses in forestry, with the exception of economics and statistics. Still motivated to do my best by my fear of failure, I was able to do well in all my courses, even economics and statistics, through diligent study. But I was also beginning to think that I might be a teacher, even a professor, one day and wanted to learn what all my courses were about.

Forestry is a difficult program of study, requiring courses in biology, botany, chemistry, zoology, ecology, dendrology, economics, soils, hydrology, algebra, analytical geometry, calculus and statistics, as well as tough courses in forest management. There was also a 10-week "summer camp" that I enrolled in between my junior and senior years where we studied surveying, forest plants and forest measurements.

Most of the courses I had taken at Hampden-Sydney transferred to Virginia Tech, with the exception of classes such as Bible and Latin which could not be exchanged for any equivalent courses in the forestry curriculum. Even though those courses did not count toward graduation, I later realized how important those courses were in influencing my life.

The Bible courses had been very difficult, and we had a tough professor. Professor "Yahweh" McCray, as students called him (not to his face, of course) taught us to understand the historical context of the old and new testaments. In Dr. McCray's class, I learned to appreciate the moral lessons taught in the Bible. Since then, although not a strongly religious man, I have tried to live my life by Jesus' words, "Do unto others as you would have them do unto you," a valuable lesson indeed.

The Latin courses, in turn, proved to be extremely helpful in my study of all those "ology" courses, where many scientific words and terms were derived from Latin and Greek. However, because the Latin and Bible courses, plus a few others, did not transfer, it took me three more years to receive my Bachelor of Science in forest management from Virginia Tech.

I did well academically at Virginia Tech, and when I graduated in 1963, I was first in my forestry class. It was a small class with about 30 students, but I was proud of my accomplishment. I believe that learning how to study at Hampden-Sydney served me well at Virginia Tech and that despite being of average intelligence, I had achieved because I just worked harder than everyone I knew.

My forestry department head at Virginia Tech, Dr. John Hosner, convinced me to pursue a Master of Science in forestry with him as my major professor. I agreed and began a program of study to determine the relationship between the growth of yellow poplar, a valuable hardwood species, and soil-mapping units. In other words,

I wanted to know if yellow poplar trees grow better on some soils than others, and if so, how much better? I published the results of my research in the *Journal of Forestry* and received the Massey Award as the outstanding graduate student in the Forestry and Wildlife Department in 1965. I enjoyed the thrill of being published in a refereed, or peer-reviewed, journal for the first time.

Fishing and forestry

EVEN DURING GRADUATE SCHOOL, fishing was still a big part of my life. In addition to fishing on my home waters of the Cowpasture and Calfpasture rivers, I fished Craigs Creek and small trout streams near my hometown on weekends and holidays when I could get home. I also occasionally fished the beautiful New River, a river recognized by geologists as the second oldest river in the world, near Blacksburg, Virginia, the home of Virginia Tech. The New River is generally regarded as the best smallmouth bass river in Virginia and possibly in the entire southeastern United States. In fact, the state record smallmouth weighing eight pounds, one ounce, was caught there in 2003.

A soil scientist who worked for the Soil Conservation Service, as the Natural Resources Conservation Service was known in those days, and who I always just called Mr. Porter helped me on the field work for my thesis project and served on my graduate committee. He also took me under his wing as a fisherman and, after our field work was done, we fished together a few times at some of his favorite spots on the New River.

We caught smallmouth bass, bluegills and other small panfish on spinning lures. About 50 years later, I would go back to those same spots on the New River with my fly rod and catch smallmouth bass weighing up to three pounds.

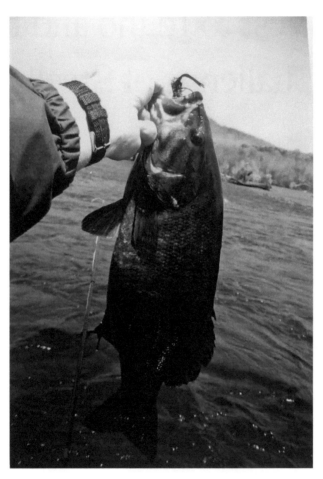

A three-pound smallmouth bass I caught on a fly
called "roadkill," in the New River,
50 years after I had first fished there

Chapter 8

West to Idaho and the Challenge of Steelhead

WHEN I WAS NEARING the end of my master's program, I began to explore opportunities for pursuing a Ph.D. Several of my professors at Virginia Tech advised me that I should go to the western United States to experience new forest ecosystems and broaden my perspective on life and forestry. That was good advice.

I applied to the University of Washington and the University of Idaho and was accepted by both universities. I decided on the University of Idaho for a couple of reasons. Both the University of Washington and the University of Idaho had strong reputations as good forestry schools, but the area around Moscow, Idaho, was much less densely populated than the Seattle area, always an important consideration for me. And there were fishing options to consider.

The decision to enroll in the University of Idaho to work toward a Ph.D. in forest sciences was extremely important in my life. The university led me to more deeply appreciate forestry research and university teaching, two areas of academia that would become the focus of my life for the next four decades.

Fishing opportunities, as usual, had a big influence on my choosing the University of Idaho and would continue to influence decisions throughout my life. Moscow, Idaho, was close to some good trout fishing streams, including the Clearwater River and its tributaries. These waters had runs of steelhead, an anadromous rainbow trout weighing up to 20 pounds.

Could I work on a doctorate in forest sciences, no easy task, and fish for steelhead too? I believed I could.

The University of Idaho sits in the middle of the Palouse country in northwestern Idaho. The Palouse is a rich agricultural area, chiefly known for wheat and legume crops, especially lentils. It is a beautiful region any time of the year and has a unique geomorphology, the result of windblown sediments from the Columbia River basin in eastern Washington being deposited in the area over thousands of years. The Palouse also has beautiful sunsets because of this windblown dust.

While at the University of Idaho, I lived with several other graduate students in an old farmhouse about seven miles from Moscow, near the small town of Troy, Idaho. We were all studying and conducting research in the area of natural resources. During the three years I lived there, my housemates included a couple of young men who were in forestry and others who were in fisheries, range management and wildlife management.

The old farmhouse was perfect for us — we called it the Big Meadow Creek Experiment Station because it sat close to a small creek named Big Meadow Creek, and we were all working on research projects.

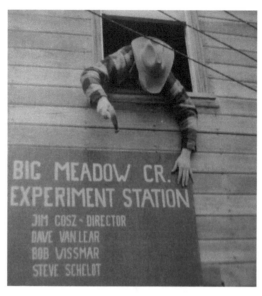

BIG MEADOW CR.
EXPERIMENT STATION
JIM COSZ - DIRECTOR
DAVE VAN LEAR
BOB VISSMAR
STEVE SCHELOT

Our farmhouse, which we called the Big Meadow Creek
Experiment Station, in Troy, Idaho

THE FARMHOUSE HAD TWO stories plus a basement where we kept a winter's worth of firewood that we cut off nearby Moscow Mountain, utilizing standing dead trees — trees that had not rotted too much to be useful for heating. The old house badly needed painting and was heated with one wood-burning stove. Despite snow blowing in through cracks in the walls during windy, blizzard-like conditions, the house was generally comfortable with ample room for four or five guys.

Those years in Idaho were a social experiment for me. I had always been a little bit of a loner, and now I was living in close quarters with three or four other guys. But all of us had similar interests academically and recreationally so we were very compatible. Besides studying and working hard on our research projects, we also hunted for deer, elk and mountain goats on weekends during hunting season. We also grew a garden, which enabled us to kill and/or grow nearly all our food. It was cheap living since we split the rent four or five ways, depending on how many of us were living in the house at the time, and we alternated driving our vehicles the seven miles to the university on a weekly basis. Although It wasn't the safest vehicle we had, Bob Wissmar's vintage 1952, 14-passenger yellow school bus was the most fun and drew the most attention when we arrived on campus in it.

One night at about 10 o'clock, our nearest neighbor, who lived about a quarter of a mile away, came to our door and asked us to help him hunt down a black bear that was tearing the trees in his apple orchard to pieces. He had summoned a local doctor who was a bear hunter and had a horse and some bear hounds. The neighbor and doctor needed a few more bodies to be stationed around the orchard, so they asked us to help. Thanks to the doctor's dogs, we were soon able to locate and tree the bear which had fled to nearby woods when he heard the dogs approaching.

The group offered to let me — I don't know why — shoot the bear out of the large pine tree it had climbed. It must have been 50 feet up that tree. With the help of a flood light the good doctor had, I aimed my .30-06 at the bear's shoulder and pulled the trigger.

All hell broke loose as the bear fell from its perch in the tree, breaking branches as it fell, woofing and snapping its teeth when it hit the ground. There were about six of us foolishly standing in a circle around that tree when the bear fell. Surrounding a wounded and angry bear is really not a good place to be. Thankfully, we scattered quickly allowing someone to get an open killing shot. I don't remember if it was me or one of my housemates who actually fired the fatal shot. Then, like now, it was all sort of a blur.

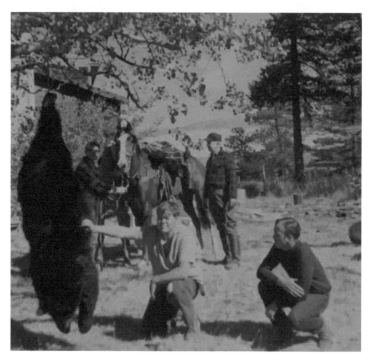

The black bear I shot because it was tearing up our
neighbor's apple trees

WHILE WE WERE ALL outdoorsmen, I was the only fisherman among the Big Meadow Creek boys. Idaho is blessed with great trout fishing, and I sampled as much of it as time would allow during the three years I was there. I had not yet been completely converted to "catch and release," so I kept the fish I caught for our supper. When I would catch a steelhead, which wasn't too often, it would feed four or five hungry young men.

I occasionally fished the upper St. Joe River which was only an hour or so away from the university and had good populations of native west slope cutthroat trout in its upper reaches. It received little fishing pressure in those days, which was always important to me. I still had the urge to stay away from crowds.

I probably inherited this "distancing" trait from my mom's side of the family. My fifth great grandmother, Mary Draper Ingles, lived with her family in a tiny village called Draper's Meadow in Virginia, the westernmost settlement in the colonies at the time, about as far away as anyone could get from civilization. In 1750 she was kidnapped by Shawnee Indians in a raid during the French and Indian War. She later escaped, making her way back home over 800 miles through an uncharted wilderness with the help of an old Dutch woman. We definitely like to be on our own.

Idaho offered lots of solitude. The North Fork Coeur d'Alene River was one of my favorite streams and was reasonably close to my research plots, so I could occasionally fish that beautiful stream after completing my field measurements.

I also fished the St. Maries, the closest trout stream to the university, about a half hour away. It was not one of the best trout streams in Idaho, but it did have a type of fish that I had never caught before — a squawfish, now called a pikeminnow by the American Fisheries Society. Pikeminnows are strong fighters on a fly rod. The ones I was able to catch were about 15- to 17-inches long.

When I arrived in Idaho, my major professor asked me to help with forestry summer camp, which was located in McCall, Idaho. This experience, he said, would help me understand and appreciate the forest ecosystems of central Idaho. While at the camp, a forest ecology professor at the university, his son and I hiked into a high mountain cirque lake — Lake 33 it was called on the U.S. Forest Service map — in the Sawtooth Mountain range of central Idaho to fish for cutthroat trout.

It was a tough hike in those days, over 60 years ago, and probably still is. There was no trail, so we just bushwhacked our way 1,600 feet up a pretty steep mountain off a Forest Service road to the saddle between two mountains and then scrambled 1,600 feet down the other side to this gorgeous little lake.

There, I first spotted a beautiful 17-inch cutthroat trout that was cruising up and down the shoreline, coming toward the high rock I was perched on. When my cast landed near him, the fish bolted and headed back the other way. After spooking it with my casts a few more times, I suddenly had the "brilliant" idea, one that any fool would have figured it out, to cast my fly out while the cutthroat was at the far end of its cruise. When the trout came back toward me this time, my fly was already on the water, so it wasn't spooked. The trout saw the fly, came up and sucked it in, and we had that fish for lunch.

That outing however, was shortened by an intense electrical storm that scared the hell out of us. We were above timberline and the lightning, booming thunder and static electricity in the atmosphere made the hair on our necks stand on end as we huddled together under an overhanging boulder. The storm didn't last long but long enough to drop the temperature 20 degrees and convince us we'd had enough fishing for that day. We were ready to get the heck off that mountain.

But no single electrical storm could dampen my devotion to fishing. The waters of Idaho sported a particularly challenging species of trout called steelhead. Steelhead trout are rainbow trout that spend several years in the ocean before coming back into their natal rivers to spawn. For me, steelhead were the hardest fish to catch because they are in the river to spawn, not eat, and they are always on the move.

I managed to only catch a dozen steelhead while I was in Idaho. All but one of those giant fish were caught on spinning gear, but one was caught on the new Fenwick fiberglass fly rod that I had just bought from a sporting goods store in Spokane. I even remember the fly — a green-butt skunk fly pattern. The year was 1968 (before graphite rods became popular), and I was so proud of that rod. It was a six-weight rod, a beautiful brown with brown and white wrappings, to which I attached a classic Pflueger Medalist reel. And I broke it in on a nine-pound steelhead. Wow! That huge steelhead was the smallest of the twelve I caught, but it proved to me that I could hook and land large, strong and explosive fish on a fly rod, a lesson I wouldn't forget.

When a fisherman feels the strike of one of those giant trout — my largest weighed 17½ pounds and was 37½ inches long — the wait is well worth it. Those fish would explode down the river, going back to the Pacific from whence they came, usually jumping a couple of times on their first downstream run and ripping line off my Mitchell 306 spinning reel. It was invigorating, after hours of standing in a lonely and cold river on a freezing winter day, to get a strike and see your line start zipping down the river with a huge fish suddenly erupting from the water.

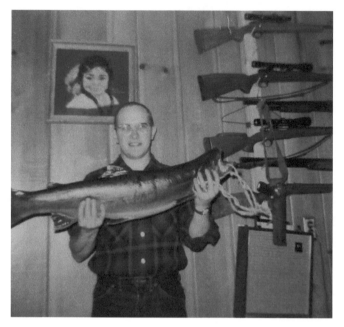

My largest steelhead, 17½ pounds and 37½ inches long

I ONCE FISHED 12 times in a row without a strike, wading in the icy Clearwater River and its tributaries with small icebergs floating down the river, my fingers numb and ice in the guides of my rod. Only a fool would fish like this, I thought! But my addiction kept me going or was it my manic, or hypomanic, behavior?

Fifty years later, I can still clearly remember each of those fish. I caught ten of those steelhead in the Clearwater River and the North Fork of the Clearwater. The other two I caught in the Lochsa and the Selway rivers, major tributaries of the Clearwater. All of those fish weighed between 12 and 15 pounds, except for that 17½-pound steelhead and the nine-pounder I caught on my fly rod.

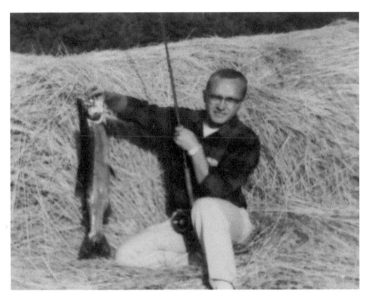

A nine-pound steelhead caught In Idaho on my new Fenwick fiberglass fly rod using a green-butt skunk fly

Chapter 9

A Deer Hunt
I Will Never Forget

THE SPARSE POPULATION AND natural beauty of Idaho made it a paradise for a graduate student/outdoorsman. I always preferred fishing to hunting, but Idaho offered me a bit of both. While I was never much of a big-game hunter, I did manage to kill three deer while in Idaho. One of my hunting trips was especially memorable. My housemates and I were camped out and hunting the breaks of the Snake River near Whitebird, Idaho. Early on the first morning of the hunt, we split up to cover more territory. I approached a large clear-cut area that, in the three or four years since the area had been cut, had become overgrown with brush.

I had stopped and watched the area for about ten minutes, when a big whitetail buck suddenly bolted from the brush about 50 yards from me. I guess he couldn't stand my being there any longer. The buck bounded away from me at a very fast pace. I dropped to one knee, steadied myself and fired. Nothing. The buck just kept bouncing through the clear-cut.

Now, the deer was at least 70 yards from me and was just about to go over the crest of the ridge. I had time for one more shot. I fired again and saw through my scope a blood spot appearing just behind his left shoulder. I knew I had hit him hard in a vulnerable spot. I ran to the top of the ridge as fast as I could and there, just on the other side, was my buck, a beautiful 10-point whitetail with a wide and perfectly symmetrical rack. A real trophy!

Excited, I sat down to rest and collect my wits. After about 15 minutes, I gutted the buck and began thinking about how I was going to get him back to camp. Since he probably weighed over 200 pounds, I would need some help.

Just as I stood up, I saw a big mule deer buck, sneaking through the brushy clear-cut, near where I had kneeled and squeezed off the shot that killed the big whitetail. This buck had not seen me, so I squatted down, placed the rifle on my knee, still shaking from the excitement of killing the big whitetail, and squeezed off a shot. He was standing absolutely still, and I had missed!

I took a deep breath to calm my nerves — I had buck fever bad by then — and my next shot hit him in the lungs. The buck went down. I ran over to confirm that he was dead and found that I had killed a big mule deer buck even larger than the whitetail buck I had just killed. He had a massive 11-point rack that was higher than it was wide. And even though I had killed two bucks in a matter of minutes, I wasn't breaking the law. It was perfectly legal to kill two deer in that part of Idaho, and I had the necessary two tags. Those two bucks would help feed the Big Meadow Creek Experiment Station boys through the long Idaho winter.

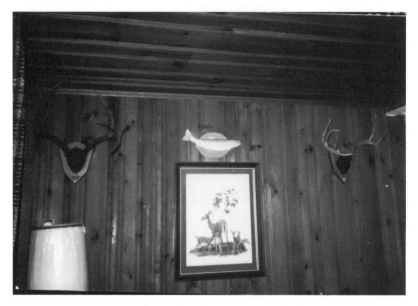

My 10-point whitetail and 11-point mule deer racks
from two deer killed within a half hour of each other
from the same clear-cut

ON A HUNT THE next year in the same area, the breaks of the Snake River, I had quite a scare. I had been scanning a large grassy, western-facing slope where the only deer cover was in a couple of draws where hardwood brush grew to a height of about 20 feet. After watching the area for a half hour or so, I decided to move farther down the slope that was steep and interspersed with large boulders.

As I was just stepping off one of those boulders, with one foot on top of the rock and the other just touching the ground below, I heard the whirring, rattling sound of a rattlesnake, about a foot away from my ankle. I knew the sound well, and I instinctively jumped downhill and away from the danger. As I jumped, I looked back in time to see the rattlesnake strike out, but thanks to quick reflexes that landed me about 10-15 feet down the slope, I was long gone. As soon as I gathered my wits, I collected some fist-sized rocks and went back up the slope to find and kill the snake that had just scared the hell out of me. But it had gotten back in the rocks, and I couldn't find it. It's probably just as well for both of us.

I decided to quit deer hunting when I left Idaho. I knew that most dedicated deer hunters hunt their whole lives and never had the luck I had in that single half hour at the clear-cut. Even I couldn't believe my good fortune. I have killed only five deer in my life, all bucks, and those two bucks were the largest deer I ever killed. Add them to the black bear that was killed after my shot dropped it from the tree, and you'd have just about all my big-game hunting. While I understand that some people seem to be driven to be big-game hunters all their lives, it's just not for me.

Chapter 10

Graduate Research With a Bit of Bass Fishing

WHILE THE RIVERS AND mountains of Idaho offered great adventures, most of my time at the University of Idaho was spent in study and research. Each morning, the Big Meadow Creek Experiment Station guys would wake up at about 6:00 a.m., eat breakfast, load up into one of our vehicles and head to school for an eight-hour day of courses and research.

My dissertation project was a study of the effects of plant-growth regulators and hormones on the growth and survival of Douglas Fir seedlings when planted in a harsh, droughty environment like that of northern Idaho. My field study was in an area known as the Athol Prairie in the northern panhandle of the state, about two hours north of the University of Idaho. In addition to the field study, my research included greenhouse and growth chamber experiments conducted at the university.

My hypothesis was that the growth and survival of planted seedlings could be improved by altering the root/shoot ratio of seedlings using plant growth hormones, at least for the first year after planting. I hypothesized that if the size of the root system could be increased while keeping the tops of seedlings from growing too much and transpiring more moisture than the roots could absorb in those first critical years, seedling survival might be enhanced. Of course, the growth could be controlled only to a certain extent. The tops of the seedlings would soon have to start growing to ensure subsequent root growth.

I found that while I was able to improve the root/shoot ratio somewhat, it unfortunately wasn't enough to improve survival of the seedlings during the two droughty summers of my experiment.

The Athol Prairie was indeed a challenging environment, both for the seedlings and for me. Summers are very hot there, with temperatures on some days reaching into the 90s. The prairie receives an average of only about one inch of rain per month in both July and August, the most stressful months for newly planted seedlings.

The seedlings in my field experiment not only suffered from severe drought conditions, they also had to contend with another threat — prairie dogs, of all things! Prairie dogs were certainly something I did not count on. They pulled many of my planted seedlings down into their underground tunnels and ate them. Thankfully I had greenhouse and laboratory studies to supplement my field experiment, so all was not lost.

And, of course, I had fishing.

I discovered a pretty little pond that was just a few hundred yards from my research plots. After completing my field measurements, I was able on a few occasions to fish the pond for an hour or two. The shoreline of the pond was covered with alder and willow bushes making it almost impossible to access parts of the pond that I wanted to fish from the bank. There was no evidence that anybody ever fished this two- to three-acre pond. With its impenetrable thickets of brush, I was sure very few people even knew the pond existed. Of course, I was drawn to it during the early-spring spawning time for bass in northern Idaho because I immediately noticed several swirls of fish that looked like bass chasing minnows or bluegills away from their spawning beds. I felt sure I could catch those fish on Rapalas, one of my favorite lures, if I could only get to them.

As they say, "Necessity is the mother of invention." My "invention" was an inner-tube boat, or a float tube or belly boat as they are now called. My float tube was made from a large truck tire inner tube onto which I attached a seat that I had sewn from a piece of canvas. I put swim fins on the feet of my stocking-foot chest waders and paddled backwards around the pond fairly easily, carrying my fishing rod and other equipment on my lap or in my fishing vest.

On my first attempt using my homemade belly boat, I had great luck and caught a six-pound largemouth bass, a large bass for such a northern latitude. That bass pulled me around the pond for a few minutes before I was able to grab it by its lower jaw and attach it to my stringer. My housemates and I ate that big boy for supper the next evening.

My Rube Goldberg-like contraption did have one major drawback. In this boat, the angler sits very low in the water and, if I leaned back just a little bit, water would come rushing into my chest waders and give me a good soaking. Since belly boats had been around for at least 20 years before my "invention" in 1967, I didn't think it would be appropriate to apply for any patents for my crude boat.

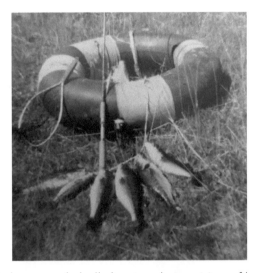

My homemade belly boat and nice string of bass
from my "secret" pond

I COMPLETED MY DISSERTATION and passed my oral exam in late spring of 1968, a few weeks too late to receive my diploma in that academic year. My Ph.D. was actually awarded by the University of Idaho in May 1969, but I was on to my next adventure by that time.

Chapter II

A Postdoc and Bass Fishing in Florida

WHEN I FINISHED MY doctoral work in Idaho in 1968, I wanted to return to the southeastern United States, see my family and enjoy the southern lifestyle again; that's the lifestyle that I had grown up with and found hard to beat. Since I was a bachelor and free to go anywhere, I applied for a postdoctoral position at the University of Florida. The position was funded by the university and about a dozen forest industries for research in the area of nutrition of slash pine plantations.

The University of Florida was a wonderful experience, allowing me to work with some of the top forest scientists in the United States and proved to be another turning point in my life.

My supervisor at the university was Dr. Wayne Smith, a superb leader and mentor to me. Dr. Smith helped me prepare for my career in many ways. Two skills he taught me in particular would prove to be important for the rest of my career: how to make presentations at scientific meetings and how to publish scientific research.

During my year at the University of Florida, I researched the effects of various soil nutrients, especially micronutrients like copper and zinc, on the physiology and growth of slash pine seedlings. During my post-doctoral program, I learned how to become a productive scientist and published two peer-reviewed papers.

I will always be grateful for all the academic and non-academic opportunities I had during my time in Florida. My best friend in Florida was an invaluable technician in the laboratory where I worked, Joel Smith, who helped all the scientists and graduate students in our lab. He was both likable and capable. In fact, I believed there was nothing he couldn't do in the lab. But more than that, he was a great friend and a pretty good bass fisherman. I did not say a "great" bass fisherman because, even today, I don't want him to get a big head. To be honest, Joel was really an excellent bass fisherman, and I owe him a great deal for showing me the ropes of fishing north Florida bass waters.

After work, Joel and I frequently fished the small, sandhill ponds around Gainesville that he knew like the back of his hand. Because he was also very familiar with several of the larger lakes and rivers in northern Florida, we had a number of fishing options. I visited his home often (his wife, Polly, was a wonderful cook), and Joel never failed to show me the 11-pound and 12-pound largemouth bass that were mounted and displayed over the mantle in his home.

Most of the time Joel and I would wade-fish those small, shallow ponds using bullhead minnows for bait. Occasionally we used artificial lures, especially plastic worms and surface plugs like the Rapala and devil's horse. I caught five large bass that year in Florida, each of which weighed about 8½ pounds and was about 25 inches long. One of those big fish is hard to forget. Joel, a friend named Jim Stephens and I were fishing Lake George, a large, shallow lake in central Florida. We had motored out into the lake in Jim's boat, anchored and got out to start wade fishing, scattering in different directions so we wouldn't compete for the same fish.

Soon after we left the boat, I spotted the sandy, white, oval shape of a bass bed which was exposed after the black muck on the bottom of the lake had been fanned out by smaller male bass. As I watched that spot, I saw the black shape of a big fish moving over the bed. I quickly put a big bullhead minnow on my hook and tossed it just past the bed, then I reeled it back until I thought my minnow would be lying in the bed. I waited.

After a few minutes, I saw the shadow of that big bass come back to the bed and stop. Then I felt a sudden sharp pull. I let her run for about ten yards, but when the bass stopped and then started up again, I struck. But I missed her. I reeled in my line and checked my hook. The bullhead minnow was gone, and there was a large fish scale impaled on the hook.

"I just missed a big ol' bass, but I hooked a scale," I shouted out to Joel and Jim. Sarcastically, they shouted back that catching scales don't count, just fish.

"Okay, just wait," I replied. "I'm going to go back there and catch that fish after I let the bed rest for a while. You'll see."

A few hours later, I went back to the area and actually caught that fish on another bullhead minnow. My Zebco De-Liar confirmed its size, 8½ pounds, a really nice bass. I hooked it, along with several smaller bass I had caught, onto my safety pin fish stringer, which was attached to a belt around my waders.

A bit later, when we met back at the boat, Joel and Jim had both caught large bass that looked to be about eight pounds each. As they held them up for me to admire, Joel said, "These are real fish, not just a fish scale. How did you do?"

"Well, let me show you something," I said and reached down for my belt stringer. When I lifted it up to show Joel and Jim a real bass, I found to my dismay that my big bass had escaped. "What the heck?" I yelled. The snap holding my big bass had come open, and she was gone. I am certain that the same fish I had missed earlier in the morning had now disappeared again!

"What big fish?" Joel asked, derisively. Of course, as I told them that I had caught that big bass, weighed it at 8½ pounds and somehow it had escaped, they just laughed and acted like I was full of it. I know they knew that I had actually caught a big bass because I wouldn't lie about something as important as that! But, of course, fishermen are known for tales of "the one that got away." This is mine, a tale of a bass that got away in quite an unusual way.

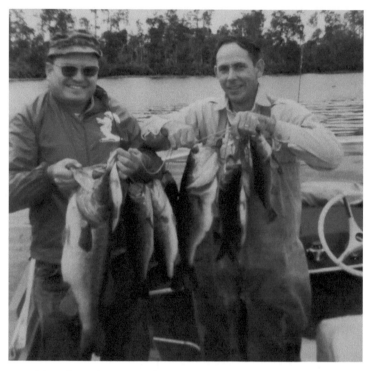

Joel Smith and Jim Stephens with bass that didn't get away
at Lake George in Florida

WHEN I ACCEPTED THE postdoctoral position at the university, I set a goal of catching a 10-pound largemouth bass during my time there. In fact, it had been a goal since I was in high school. Each of the five large bass I caught that year in Florida might have weighed at least 10 pounds if I had caught them before they had spawned. But fisheries biologists say that as bass spawn out, they lose two to three pounds of eggs.

During the year of my postdoctoral appointment, I tried hard to match at least one of those two big bass over Joel's mantle, but I was going to have to leave Florida before that goal could be accomplished.

When my postdoctoral appointment at the University of Florida ended, I accepted a position with the U.S. Forest Service in Berea, Kentucky, as a research forester working on the reclamation of coal strip mines.

When I arrived in Berea in late September 1969, I felt lucky to find a basement apartment in a very nice brick house belonging to a Mr. Boggs, who owned a grocery store in town that, to me, was eerily similar to the store my dad had operated in Clifton Forge. Berea is best known as the home of Berea College, a small liberal arts college that was established to educate mountain youth from the Appalachia region. My apartment was only a few blocks from the college and a couple of miles from the Forest Service laboratory where I worked.

My job in Berea would prove to be difficult. Fortunately for me, I had my addiction to fishing to lure me back to Florida the next year for a few days in February, before the spawn, to try my luck again at catching a 10-pound largemouth. Because of work responsibilities, my friend Joel Smith, could not fish with me the first day, but I told him that I would have to fish anyway.

"Too bad, Joel, but I'll catch a big one for you," I told him. I left Joel in the lab and found my way through the longleaf pine and scrub oak forest near Gainesville to the small pond that he had shown me the previous year.

As I waded out into the pond, I again saw the swept-out bed of a spawning bass, clearly visible where the white sandy bottom was exposed after the dark organic muck had been swept away by smaller male bass. As I watched the bed, a large dark shadow swam over it, just like that big bass I had caught and then lost on Lake George the previous year.

"My God, that was a big bass!" I thought as I quickly took a large bullhead minnow from my bait bucket, hooked it through the lips and cast it about five feet beyond the bed. I slowly pulled the minnow back until I thought it was sitting on the bed and waited.

After a few minutes, there was a tug on my line, and it started to move away, a hard and steady pull. I let the fish run and run. When it stopped, I leaned forward, reeled in the slack line and struck hard. Nothing. But off to my left a big fish rolled on the surface.

Was that my fish? I was certain it was! That fish had eaten my minnow and run straight away from me. When it passed some rushes sticking out of the water, it took a hard left. I hadn't realized this sudden change of direction when I first struck, but now I knew, so I reeled up more slack and struck again. This time I had it.

The bass wallowed on the surface and headed toward an old barbed-wire fence that stretched across that end of the pond. If it got tangled in that, I would lose it for sure. Finally, I was able to put the brakes on the bass just before it got to the fence. It was too heavy to jump clear of the surface of the water, but after a few more wallows on the surface, I was able to grab it by the lower jaw and haul it to the bank. The heft told me this was likely my elusive 10-pound bass.

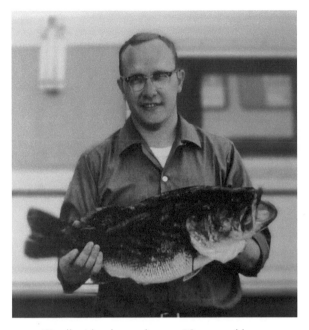

Finally, I had caught my 10-pound bass

MY ZEBCO DE-LIAR SAID the bass weighed 10½ pounds! Back at our lab, Joel weighed it at 10 pounds, 6 ounces on the lab's official scales. I could now cross that goal of catching a 10-pound bass off my bucket list.

Chapter 12

Strip Mining in Kentucky

MY JOB WITH THE U.S. Forest Service was not proving to be as productive as my fishing, however.

The mission of our research unit was to find the best methods to reclaim strip-mined lands after the underlying coal seam has been removed. Strip mining involves the removal of rock and soil that lie above nearly horizontal beds of coal which, in the mountains of eastern Kentucky, ranged from about two- to five-feet thick.

The layers of rock and soil lying over these seams of coal could be more than 50 feet deep. This overburden, as those layers are called, is removed by blasting it with powerful explosives then scooping away the rock and soil using huge draglines. The exposed coal is then carried away in gigantic trucks.

Our team of researchers included a hydrologist, a mechanical engineer, a range scientist and me, a research forester, along with several technicians and a secretary. Our team was tasked with finding methods to reduce the environmental impacts of mining by using techniques to physically manipulate the overburden in order to reduce erosion, while identifying plants, from grasses to shrubs to tree species, that could tolerate the harsh conditions. The overall effect was to stabilize these spoil banks and provide habitat for wildlife.

Needless to say, spoil banks were often either acid, droughty, compacted, or all of these and very difficult to reclaim. In eastern Kentucky, these spoil banks were also on precipitous slopes which meant that until they could be successfully revegetated, if ever, they were sources of excessive erosion and sedimentation of streams draining the steep mountain terrain. Besides negatively impacting aquatic life, spoil banks were generally poor wildlife habitat because of sparse vegetative cover and low plant diversity.

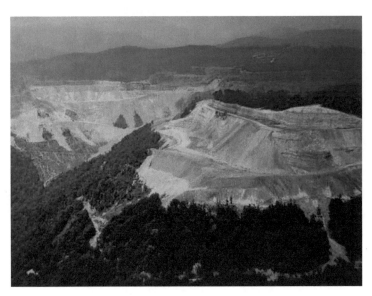

Strip mining in the steep slopes of Appalachia causes severe erosion and sedimentation of streams.

OUR TEAM OF RESEARCHERS and technicians worked diligently to document the impacts of strip mining on the environment and to find and demonstrate successful methods of reclamation. My research there dealt with the effects of various fertilizers and lime on growth of plants used in reclamation efforts, plant species such as black locust, love grass and many others. However, my impression of our efforts was that they were like putting a band-aid on a chainsaw injury. I found my time in Kentucky to be frustrating.

In my mind, there was no way our efforts, as well intentioned as they were, could compensate for the extreme environmental damage that strip mining and mountaintop mining was doing to Appalachian mountain ecosystems. I believed that our publications showing modest success in reclamation efforts were being used by surface-mining companies as false advertisements about the success of their efforts to reclaim spoil banks. Because I wanted no part of that message, after about a year in Berea I was on the lookout for a way out of Kentucky.

But before I left Kentucky, I would fish.

A good friend, Phil Marcum, who was a technician in our lab, and I made a trip to the Lynch River in hopes of catching a muskellunge, or "muskie," as the fish is usually called. I had never even fished for the species, much less caught one, but we had recently read reports in the Lexington newspaper that there were indeed muskies in that river.

Phil and I towed my small bass boat to a U.S. Forest Service boat ramp on the Lynch River one September weekend in 1970. Often called the fish of 1,000 casts, or even 10,000 casts, we knew the muskie would be difficult to catch, but we were anxious to give it a try.

Phil and I were using large Rapala-type lures. After fishing several hours with no hits, I finally had a savage strike. It was a muskie, but only about 24-inches long. They had to be 40 inches to be legal at the time, so I admired and then released the only muskie I have ever caught. As a dedicated fisherman, I can claim that catch as the highlight of my fishing in Kentucky. It's no wonder I felt depressed much of my time in Kentucky. Even though I had made some good friends there, I was lonely, didn't like my job and my fishing opportunities were scarce. Not a good combination of factors for me.

What my job in Kentucky did make me appreciate in a very real way was the interrelationships among the various components of the environment and how man's abuse of technology can overwhelm the environment's ability to mitigate that abuse. In college, I had studied relations among environmental components, such as forest, soil, wildlife and water, and how man's activities interact with them. But it took Kentucky and strip mining for me to take that knowledge to my heart.

Chapter 13

A Full Life

AFTER TWO YEARS IN Kentucky, I reached the next major turning point in my life in 1971. It came in the form of a phone call from the head of the Department of Forestry, now called the Department of Forestry and Environmental Conservation, at Clemson University in Clemson, South Carolina.

Dr. Robert Allen invited me to the university to interview for a teaching/research position on the faculty. Even today, I am not sure how he got my name; I believe that he may have learned about me from my major professor at Virginia Tech, Dr. John Hosner, who I am sure I could have counted on for a good recommendation. The invitation was unusual to be sure. In normal procedure, I would have had to make a formal application for the job. While I hadn't planned for this big break, I jumped at the opportunity.

Dr. Allen was searching for a professor of silviculture. And so I drove southeast from Berea to Clemson for an interview, which lasted two days. Although I thought I had aced the interview, Dr. Allen did not make any commitment to me when I left. I later came to know that he was a man of few words.

I liked so much what I saw during the interview, that I did not submit any reimbursement expenses for travel, motel and food to Dr. Allen when the interview was over. I guess I thought that not asking for reimbursement would make the selection committee look a little more favorably on me. I really wanted this job.

A few days later I received a check reimbursing me for my interview expenses, plus an offer for the associate professor position. The offer was for $16,600 per year. While it does not sound like much money now, in 1971 it sounded good to me. In fact, it was $500 more than I was making with the U.S. Forest Service in Kentucky. I gladly accepted his offer — one of the luckiest breaks of my life — and thus began my 35 years at Clemson teaching silviculture, a subject I loved teaching. When my appointment began, I was to split my time equally: 50 percent teaching and 50 percent research. Over the last two decades of my career at Clemson my work shifted to about 30 percent teaching and 70 percent research.

Most people don't know what silviculture is, but some of us call silviculture the "heartbeat of forestry" because it is so fundamental to the practice of forestry. It is applied forest ecology, a component of the broader concept of forest management. Silviculture is about the physical manipulation of forest stands, using practices such as thinning, harvesting, prescribed burning and other tools, to ensure that the entire forest produces the benefits desired by the landowner, whether it be private landowners or the federal government.

Through silviculture, the forest produces products and values such as wood products, wildlife habitat, quality water or recreational opportunities. Even if a forest owner simply wants certain areas to be preserved with no active treatments applied, just protection, silviculture is still involved. In that case nature instead of man will make the changes in the stand, either gradually through succession or suddenly via a major disturbance.

The public generally doesn't think much about the many economic benefits from forests, except perhaps in lumber or paper production. People generally understand that forests are an important component of their environment, beautiful to look at as well as providing habitat for wildlife, preventing soil erosion, reducing air pollution, storing carbon, producing the oxygen we breath, providing recreational opportunities and supplying timber and pulpwood for our lumber and paper. They don't really care about everything that is necessary to make forests more productive or technical concepts such as marginal rates of return, basal area, silvicultural systems and stocking guidelines.

That's all encompassed in silviculture. It ensures that forests produce whatever we value: economic benefits, recreational opportunities or environmental betterment. It shapes the forests we see and know.

My first silvicultural research project when I came to Clemson was a study of the application of the shelterwood method, a stand regeneration method that involves the removal of about half of the mature overstory trees to naturally regenerate desired species on high-quality Piedmont sites. My research evolved over my career to include studies on nutrient cycling, the role of fire in forest ecosystems, root systems of mature forest trees, and other areas related to silviculture.

Time for a turn for the better

By 1978 I HAD been a bachelor so long that I had begun to think that marriage was not for me. I was 37 years old, a chaired full professor at Clemson University and had not had any real serious girlfriends for a long time, if I ever. Perhaps, I thought, I'm just not good marriage material and no woman would want to marry me. I'd had that sad thought periodically for some years.

I don't know why I thought that I was not marriage material. I had a great job, was (at least in my mind) fairly good looking. I loved my family and my old basset hound, Doc, who was my best friend at the time. Truthfully, I suspect my major handicap with women was the fact that I was very shy. In high school when the teacher would call on me or when a girl would speak to me, I would blush deeply. I couldn't help it.

By my 30's, I was not so extremely shy, but by then it seemed that all the women I might have been interested in were already "taken." So, I just resolved to be a bachelor and try to be happy with my life as it was. It was a good life.

After my dad died, Mom had tried to live in our family home, but her physical health would not allow that. For one thing, she was not strong enough to go down into the basement and put coal in the coal-fired furnace that was used to heat the house.

Since I was a bachelor and had a good job with Clemson University, I urged her to sell the house and come live with me. A year later, in 1977, we bought a house in Pendleton, South Carolina, and moved in — just Mom, Doc and me.

Mom lived with me for two years and ultimately was the first to meet the best turning point in my life.

In 1977 a new neighbor from across the street, Carolyn Thompson stopped by the house while I was attending a forest soils conference in Albuquerque, New Mexico. She told my mom she was collecting donations in the neighborhood for a PTA school project. When my mom invited Carolyn in, they became immediate friends and wound up talking for hours about the tough times they were both going through — my mom dealing with Dad's suicide and Carolyn in the middle of a divorce.

One afternoon not long afterwards, Doc and I were out in the front yard of our new house, just checking it out. That's when Doc decided to take matters in his own hands, I mean paws, to find me a woman before it was too late. Doc glanced across the street and saw a beautiful young lady in a yellow jumpsuit and her pretty eight-year-old daughter walking down the sidewalk.

Before I could scream "No!" Doc bolted off, running across the street at breakneck speed — at least breakneck speed for a basset with a lame front leg — to check out these two ladies. They were as infatuated with Doc as he was with them. I followed Doc in short order and introduced myself. They told me they lived in the house just across the street. Carolyn, the lady in the yellow jumpsuit, also told me she was going through a messy divorce and had two children, her daughter, Melanie, and son, Chris.

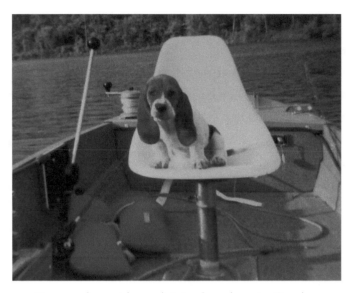

Doc, my basset hound, introduced me to Carolyn

CAN YOU BELIEVE IT? After 37 years, here was the woman of my dreams, and she was just across the street from me — and she would soon be divorced!

I had never been too sure about "love at first sight" but, darn, I believe it now. I was smitten with Carolyn on that first occasion and was able to work up the nerve to call her a few days later to ask her to have dinner with me. But doggone it! She said she would love to go, but her divorce was not yet final, so she didn't feel like she should accept my offer. She said she would let me know when her divorce became final. I was impressed by her principles, although disappointed to be sure.

About a month later, we ran into each other again at the Forestry Club's Christmas tree lot. Her 15-year-old son Chris spotted me — probably because I was driving my new white Mustang. Carolyn and Chris came over to me, and we started a conversation. I always found her so easy to talk to. Unfortunately, she told me her divorce was still not final.

The next time I saw Carolyn, she was walking around the block, this time by herself. Glory be! She quickly told me her divorce was now final, and I called her the next day and asked her to have dinner with me at a nice Mexican restaurant in Greenville, South Carolina. She said, "Yes," so we went to El Matador that Saturday night.

We instantly hit it off and talked — and talked — so long after we finished eating that the management almost had to run us out of the building when closing time approached. We had so much to learn about each other, and I thought she was so beautiful and sweet.

We had a nine-month courtship and, as the late Johnny Cash sang in his song "Ring of Fire," the flame burned higher. We were so compatible that we decided to get married in December 1978.

After a small wedding with just our immediate families, we took our honeymoon on the Outer Banks of North Carolina and in the Shenandoah Valley of Virginia, during Clemson's Christmas break.

With Carolyn, her two children, Doc, her little dachshund JJ and me in her nice but modest-sized house, we did not have room for Mom. Thankfully, my sister, Kitty, who was teaching German in Virginia Beach and unmarried at the time, agreed to move down to Clemson and live with Mom in the house Mom, Doc and I had previously shared.

The change worked well for all of us. I think Kitty was a little burned out after teaching for 25 years and was looking for a new life. She was able to get a job as a secretary in the Department of Parks, Recreation and Tourism at Clemson University. Two years later, she fell in love with and married Bill Neckerman, a man who was very much like her in his attitudes and likes and dislikes. I guess that proved that if you wanted to get married, the thing to do was move in with Mom or have Mom move in with you! At least it worked for Kitty and me.

Mom continued to live with Kitty and Bill for the next 16 years, until her death at age 84. I deeply appreciate what Kitty and Bill did for Mom, but I never got the impression that Mom was very happy in that situation. Mom would never complain because as I have said, she was a stoic little lady.

My sister, Kitty, was a very driven person and had little tolerance of anything that was not precise and well defined. She had long worked with a demanding teaching schedule, but she may also have had a touch of bipolar disorder. However, despite being rather dogmatic, Kitty loved her family and would do anything to help us.

But for me in 1978, it was wonderful to be so in love. I had come to the most important turning point in my life — meeting my wife Carolyn. At age 37 fate had brought this wonderful woman to the house across the street, and my old basset hound Doc had introduced us. Can you believe that?

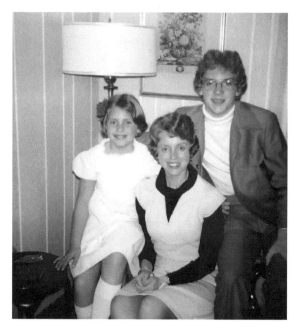

Melanie, Carolyn and Chris, my new family

Now, IN ADDITION TO my professorship and hobbies, I settled into life at Clemson as a husband to Carolyn and as a father to Chris and Melanie.

Life as a chaired professor

DURING MY SECOND YEAR at Clemson, I had inherited from a retiring professor another class called Forest Protection, a course about defending forests against wildfire, insects and disease. By 1973, I was teaching two courses, both in the spring semester, beginning a silvicultural research program and looking for graduate students to mentor.

Over time, I supervised the programs of 45 graduate students. While our department did not have a doctoral program until about midway through my career, I was fortunate enough to supervise 10 of those graduate students through their doctoral program. I also developed a graduate course called Forest Site Capability and served on the committees of at least 60 other graduate students who were working toward degrees with other professors.

Teaching undergraduates was a top priority of mine, too. In my career, I probably taught about 1,000 undergraduate students, trying my best to help them understand the concepts of silviculture and forest protection, while being a good role model and mentor. My goal was never to try to overwhelm or impress students with "high-falutin'" terminology, but to explain complex technical terms and concepts with words that they could take to heart.

I never forget the words of Havilah Babcock, a famous mid-1900s South Carolina outdoor author and chair of the English department at the University of South Carolina. When asked the secret to a successful writing career, Babcock said, "First, find a subject worth writing about, then make it simple, then make it clear and then take it to the heart." While I may have paraphrased Dr. Babcock a bit, I have learned that the last part of his statement is the hardest, but it is the part I have most enjoyed trying to do.

Along with my teaching responsibilities, research was always a major part of my academic life, accounting for from 50 to 70 percent of my duties. Many of my studies were conducted on the 17,500-acre Clemson Experimental Forest, which is practically adjacent to campus, an advantage that few, if any, other universities have.

Throughout my career at Clemson, I tried to establish a solid reputation as a forest scientist and professor, not only for myself and my students, but for the forestry department and university, both of which I had grown to love. While I was very diligent in attempting to fulfill my teaching and research responsibilities, I was also extremely fortunate to have wonderful graduate students and technicians who helped me with important research projects.

Most of my early studies involved the manipulation of forest stands and the effects of those manipulations on various components of the environment. My graduate students and I cooperated with the U.S. Forest Service's Coweeta Hydrologic Laboratory, a world-renowned forest research laboratory, on several studies, the first of which was to determine the effects of prescribed fire and timber harvesting on water quality and nutrient cycling in loblolly pine stands in the Piedmont.

In a later study with the Coweeta lab, my doctoral student, Craig Hedman, determined loadings of coarse woody debris, i.e., tree boles, root wads and branches, an important component of aquatic habitats, in Southern Appalachian streams bordered by forests ranging in age from early successional to old growth. His work has been widely cited in scientific literature.

Most of the silvicultural research projects later in my career related to the uses and effects of prescribed fire on hardwood forest ecosystems, especially to encourage oak regeneration. Using fire in hardwood forests was an area in which few other fire scientists dared to tread. The use of fire in hardwood stands had long been considered taboo by most foresters. That view is not universally held today, due, in part, to our efforts,

Another study focused on the root systems of mature loblolly pine trees. Although there have been many studies of the root systems of pine seedlings, there have been relatively few studies of the root systems of mature pine trees because of the difficulty dealing with the clay soils of the Piedmont. Yet root systems are so important to the functioning of forest ecosystems. Undeterred, one of my graduate students, Peter Kapeluck, took on this task and actually excavated the root systems of mature loblolly pine trees and then calculated their biomass and carbon content.

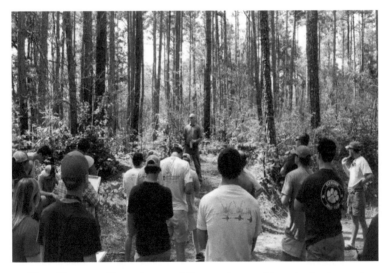

The Clemson Experimental Forest is used by students and faculty for teaching, research and demonstration, as well as for recreation.

IN YET ANOTHER RESEARCH project, Jim Abercrombie, assistant district ranger for the Sumter National Forest, developed a shelterwood-burn technique to regenerate mixed pine and hardwood stands in the South Carolina mountains. I was honored to write scientific papers describing Jim's novel method.

In 2005, W.D. Carroll, P.R. Kapeluck and I, along with Rhett Johnson, co-founder of the Longleaf Alliance, published a paper about the history and restoration of the longleaf pine-grassland ecosystem, an ecosystem that had been in sharp decline over the past century. Happily, longleaf pine is making a gradual but steady comeback, thanks to the work of the Longleaf Alliance.

Other studies with U.S. Forest Service and university scientists during my career, included cooperative projects with investigators at Oak Ridge, Tennessee, the University of Nevada, the University of Washington, the University of Florida and other institutions.

Because of cooperative efforts with graduate students, technicians and peers, I also have been able to research topics beyond my field of silviculture. Some of these "extracurricular" research projects related to the loading of coarse woody debris (boles, branches and root wads of fallen trees) in mountain streams; the effects of beaver on trout habitat in the Southern Appalachians; and the movement and home range of spawning brown trout in the Chattooga River.

While these projects were outside the realm of traditional silviculture, all seemed to involve streams and trout. Certainly, that is no coincidence! I liked to think of myself as a serious angler who never put his teaching and research responsibilities on the back burner. The two just seemed to go arm-in-arm.

Chapter 14

Bass and Trout Fishing in South Carolina

DESPITE A HEAVY LOAD of teaching and research, I still found time to fish; it seemed to me that I had to. I bought three small bass boats while working at Clemson over 35 years. How could I resist? The Clemson campus lies along the shores of Lake Hartwell, a 50,000-acre lake. Here and at other nearby lakes, I became a serious bass fisherman.

Soon after my arrival at Clemson, I had made friends with Willy Williams and Ken Sterling, graduate students in forestry who both loved to fish. The three of us would frequently fish together for large-mouth bass. We even joined BASS, the Bass Anglers Sportsman Society, not to become tournament fishermen, but believing that we could get valuable information from professional bass fishermen that would make us more successful in our bass-fishing endeavors.

A few years into our friendship, Willy became the forestry department's biometrician. In that role, he was a great help to me with statistical analyses and experimental design in my research projects.

To this day, Willy is a great friend. He and I fished for largemouth bass and hybrid bass (a cross between striped bass and white bass) in Lake Hartwell and Lake Keowee for many years. We caught many largemouths and hybrids in the two-pound class, plus a few in the four- to eight-pound class.

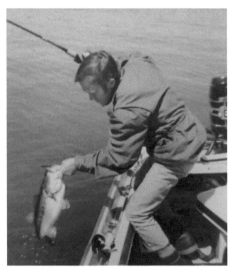

Willy landing an 8½-pound bass

WE ALSO FISHED LAKE Jocassee, a manmade lake, as it was filling up in the early 1970s. Early one October morning, fishing with Willy, I hooked and landed a huge brown trout that weighed 8½ pounds, even after it had spewed out two to three pounds of eggs onto the bottom of my boat. I feel sure that trout would have weighed ten pounds if I had weighed her before she released her eggs. I never dreamed that I would catch a brown trout that big — the largest brown trout I ever caught in Lake Jocassee.

In later years on Jocassee I would go on to catch several brown trout in the five-pound range on five-inch Rapalas, fishing from the bank near the boat ramp before the sun came up. But nothing came close to the 8½-pound monster, which was really a 10-pounder when Willy first netted it.

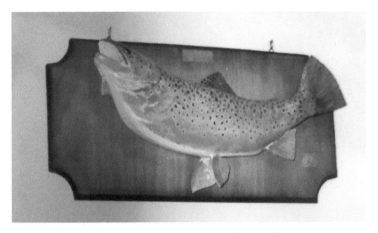

My 8½-pound brown trout caught from Lake Jocassee

ON ANOTHER FALL MORNING at Lake Jocassee, I heard huge splashes as big brown trout came to the surface in the dark. I couldn't be sure why they were splashing on the surface; were they feeding or was it some spawning behavior? Whatever their reason, I hooked one when I cast to a splash, but couldn't hold the fish as it dived to the bottom. It snapped my 6-pound test line before I could loosen my drag and was gone in a few seconds. The fish felt like a monster, maybe bigger than my 10-pounder --- oops, I'm sorry, fishermen can't help themselves. We just have to round up.

On one late spring weekend Willy and I decided to fish Lake Se-
cession, a 1,500-acre lake in Abbeville County, which we heard had
some very large bass. We had fished for several hours, using plastic
worms, when I felt some brush on the bottom.

"Willy," I told him, "there is some brush where I just cast. Throw
your worm over there. Might be a good bass there."

When Willy did, he soon had a tap. A bass was checking out his
plastic worm. When it started to run, Willy set the hook and was
onto a big bass. The fish came to the surface and tried to jump but
could only wallow on the surface. That bass had the biggest mouth
of any bass I had ever seen, and remember, I had seen Joel Smith's
mounted 12-pound bass! Based on the size of its mouth, I believed
this fish would weigh at least 12 or 13 pounds. A minute or two later,
when Willy landed the fish and weighed it on my Zebco De-Liar, it
weighed only about 8½ pounds. It was 27½-inches long, but it was a
long and skinny old bass instead of a chunky pre-spawn bass.

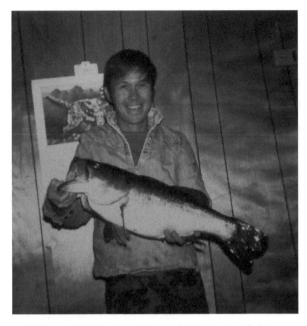

Willy and his huge 27½-inch largemouth bass

APPARENTLY, THE BASS HAD recently spawned and must have been very old. Turns out that bass lose weight when they become very old. In fact, the South Carolina Department of Natural Resources once recorded a largemouth bass that was 17 years old but weighed only four pounds. If Willy's bass had been in prime condition before spawning and a little younger, I'm sure it would have been one of the largest bass caught in South Carolina that year.

Quite a few of my students, along with those of some other professors, were bitten by the trout fishing "bug" while they were working with me on their graduate degrees at Clemson. Two of them, Rick Myers and Kyle Burrell, were bitten quite hard!

Rick, who received his Ph.D. under my direction in the early 1990s, became a lifelong friend. He and I have fished together occasionally from the time he was an undergraduate up to last year.

One of Rick's great fishing accomplishments is that he established and maintains the Crappie Rodeo, a fishing "club" that has met in South Carolina every spring for 40 straight years, until Covid-19 stopped it in 2020. The rodeo is made up of approximately 20 to 30 of Rick's good friends (including his former classmate the provost of Clemson University) who get together each spring and fish for crappie over a long weekend. I am so proud of Rick because he is the Stewardship Manager for Virginia's Natural Areas Program, putting most of his energy into conservation of special places in Virginia, but still finds time to be an angler. I guess in that sense, he reminds me of me.

Kyle Burrell, my other graduate student with a bad case of the fishing virus, came to Clemson already infected with the bug. Kyle had been shepherded through his teenage years by the Rabun Chapter of Trout Unlimited in Clayton, Georgia, his hometown. The folks in that chapter had taught him practically everything about fly fishing, and he was an expert fly fisherman by the time he came to the university to study for a master's degree.

At about the same time that Kyle arrived, the U.S. Forest Service wanted a study done about brown trout migration during the spawning season in the Chattooga River. Of course, I am not a fisheries biologist, but I had worked closely with the Andrew Pickens Ranger District of the Sumter National Forest on several silvicultural studies and was well acquainted with their regional trout biologist, Monte Seehorn. They also knew that my new graduate student was a serious trout fisherman who had practically been raised on the Chattooga River.

Perhaps based on my reputation, Kyles's knowledge and the fact that I was a serious trout fisherman, the U.S. Forest Service was confident that I could do the study and give them the information they wanted. They awarded us the study.

Kyle surgically implanted radio transmitters in adult brown trout and, using telemetry, tracked the fish over a one-year period as they migrated upstream in the fall to spawn and returned downstream to the area they had come from before spawning. To ensure our efforts would be legitimate and accepted by the scientific community, we put two fisheries biologists on Kyle's graduate committee, one from Clemson, Dr. Jeff Isely, and one from the U.S. Forest Service, Dr. Andy Dolloff, who was stationed at Virginia Tech.

The U.S. Forest Service and their fisheries people were pleased with how we conducted the study and its results. In 2000, Kyle's study was published in the *Transactions of the American Fisheries Society*, and we presented the results of our study at several meetings, including one at a Forestry-Fisheries Conference in Alberta, Canada in 1994. Never missing an opportunity to fish, we hired a guide while at the conference and floated the Bow River, a river famous for its big trout.

It was late April, and the river was still very cold from a long winter. Our guide, Mike Guinn, told us that we were too early for good fishing, but, he said, we might want to come back when the river had warmed a bit. "Ha-ha, Mike!" We told him that as nice as that would be, our lives didn't work that way. We couldn't just leave South Carolina anytime we would like to fish a river in Alberta, Canada, 3,000 miles away.

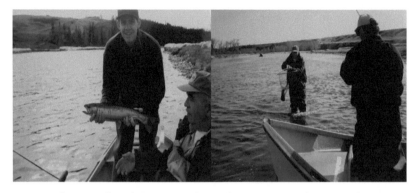

Kyle Burrell with his 20-inch rainbow trout and our guide,
Mike Guinn, netting mine on the Bow River in Canada

IN SPITE OF MIKE's warning about the fishing, we floated the river and nearly froze our rear ends off. However, we were able to catch about 20 trout, including two, 20-inch rainbows, one for Kyle and one for me. But catching 20 trout in about seven hours of fishing was pretty slow fishing for us. And it was very, very cold; there was still snow on the banks of the river in places. I told Mike that I hoped to get back to the Bow one day when the weather was more favorable. I did, but it would be ten years later.

After Kyle completed his Master of Science, he became a fishing guide, splitting his time between the Green River in Wyoming and the Chattahoochee River in Georgia. Now, when he is not guiding, Kyle works as a forestry consulting technician.

Chapter 15

Finding Balance

MY CAREER AT CLEMSON University was productive in many ways. During my time there, I published over 150 research and technical papers, as many as, or perhaps more than, any other pure silviculturist in the country. During the late 1980s, I was also supervising the programs of twelve graduate students, four of whom I had taken on when another professor left. It seemed that a large number of students wanted to work with me for master and doctoral degrees. I was also teaching two undergraduate courses and leading our Trout Unlimited chapter's stream and brook trout restoration projects. I was operating at a manic pace.

After intense periods of high productivity like this, I would often slide into a mild depression for a week or two. Throughout my whole career I never told anybody about my mood swings, knowing the stigma that mental illness has in our society. I blamed my thoughts on mild bipolar disorder, but I didn't consider them serious enough to see a doctor. I just plowed through.

Eventually my fear of failure, a strong work ethic, a loving wife and fishing would help me come out of it. Fishing always seemed necessary to help keep me happy and emotionally stable.

And fish I did.

Fortunately for my addiction to fly fishing, which had been put on hold for the three years I was in Florida and Kentucky, I did not teach in the fall semesters at Clemson, so I could take almost annual trips to the Rockies. I tried to plan these around professional conferences or meetings where I presented my research or participated in other ways. Anywhere west of the Mississippi River was close enough to the Rockies for me, and I would take a few days, maybe even a week, of annual leave before or after my meeting, rent a car and fish the streams of Yellowstone again or head to other famous streams in the Rockies I had read about since I was a kid. Carolyn often went with me. What a life!

Carolyn loved the Rockies almost as much as I did. Yellowstone National Park was always our favorite destination. We often stayed in the little tourist town of West Yellowstone where Carolyn could shop, read or just sleep in, while I could readily fish the nearby Madison, Firehole or Gibbon rivers in the mornings. I would sometimes fish one of the park's less-famous small streams, like Iron, Grayling or Duck creeks, where I would seldom see another angler. Then, I would come back to our motel, pick up Carolyn and tour the park with her in the afternoon. Sometimes, we would drive around the figure-eight loop in the park in the afternoon, enjoying the animals, the geyser basins and the scenery, with occasional stops for me to fish a bit.

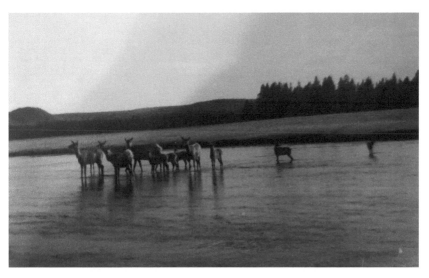

A herd of elk I saw while fishing the Firehole River

WE NEVER TIRED OF seeing the wildlife in Yellowstone, notably the herds of elk and bison, the occasional grizzly and wolf, bald eagles, geese and ducks, and the magnificent scenery too, even after more than 30 times visiting the park together. We often went into the park late in the evening when bull elk would be bugling to warn other bulls that these ladies were his and "you guys had better stay away unless you wanted a hell of a fight."

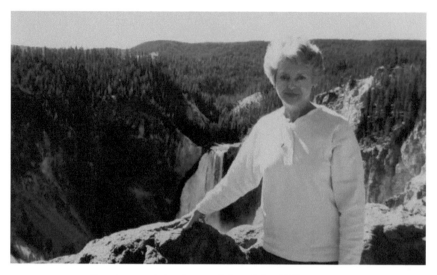

Carolyn and the lower falls of the Yellowstone

FLY FISHING MADE ME feel better mentally and physically. A few days of fly fishing in a clear trout stream in the northern Rockies in September or October did wonders for my state of mind.

While wading knee- or waist-deep in a river in Yellowstone, I would occasionally hear a bull elk bugling in the evening. I once witnessed a bald eagle swoosh down from a snag and scoop up, or try to scoop up, a large trout from the Madison River. This time the trout, which appeared to be about five pounds, was too large for the eagle to fly away with, although it tried. Instead, the eagle just sat in the water and used its wings to paddle itself and its fish to the shore, where it was able to hop up on the bank and have lunch, a sight I'll never forget. It's amazing what you can see and hear during 50-plus years of fishing in the Rocky Mountains.

Lasting impressions also remain with me of scenery framed by the dark green foliage of conifers, the golden-yellow leaves of cottonwoods and aspen, and the gin-clear waters of trout streams.

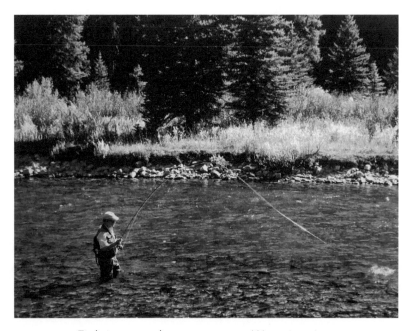

Fighting a cutthroat trout on a Wyoming river

Chapter 16

A Yellowstone Trip to Remember

ONE OF MY FONDEST memories of fly fishing in Yellowstone country centers around the largest trout I ever caught there. In September 1986, my good friend, Rick Myers, and I took annual leave from Clemson University to fish the streams of Yellowstone country for a solid week.

On this particular day, we were on the Madison River outside the park, about a mile below Reynolds Bridge. Rick was about 100 yards below me and out of sight. The water was very swift, and I was wade-fishing upstream, close to the bank. As I was approaching a frothy pocket, deeper than most I had seen that morning, with a large dead cottonwood tree lying partially submerged along the shore, I thought, "There's got to be a big fish here."

Using a #4 olive girdle bug, I made a short cast into the foaming pocket. As soon as the fly hit the water, a huge brown trout charged up from below, hitting the girdle bug hard as it leaped horizontally from the water. I struck and felt the weight of the big trout before it hit the water again, but suddenly my girdle bug came right back at me. The big fish was gone in an instant. I had just lost the biggest trout I ever hooked, or almost hooked, in Yellowstone country, even though I thought I had done everything right. What a bummer!

When Rick and I met a little later for our shore lunch, I complained about what had happened. He was not too sympathetic, probably thinking this was just one more of the many fish tales he had heard from me.

"Okay, wise guy, I'll show you," I told him. "I'm going back there this afternoon and catch that fish. Be ready to eat your words." Rick loved to joke with me and I with him.

Several hours later, I was approaching that same piece of pocket water, just as before. When I was about 30 yards from where I had previously missed the big brown, a drift boat with two anglers came within view. They were on the other side of the river, but suddenly the oarsman began rowing toward the middle. They got out of the boat, and one angler held it in place beside a large boulder while the other waded closer and began casting a large streamer fly into the foaming pocket water where I had missed "my" fish.

I would be willing to bet that angler had hooked and missed "my" fish before, or perhaps caught and released it. After a half dozen or so casts, with no strikes, they got back into their boat and floated on down the river. I guess the hex I was putting on him in my mind worked.

I let the pocket rest for about 15 minutes, then continued to stealthily approach the spot where I had missed the big one. When I was about 30 feet below the pocket, I let the current load my rod behind me — no false casting to spook the fish. I flipped my fly toward the frothy pocket water. Darn, my fly and the tip of my leader wrapped around a limb of that dead cottonwood tree. I couldn't shake it loose so I was forced to wade up to where I could use the tip of my rod to free the fly. Thoroughly disgusted, I assumed that trout was not going to be caught this day by me.

While I was standing there, fuming, waist deep in the river, I casually flipped my fly about 10 feet into a nearby pocket of foaming water. Wham! Another hard strike, and this time I had him. It was a very big trout, and I was sure it was the same one I had missed earlier in the day. He made a beeline for the dead cottonwood lying along the bank. No doubt he had escaped previous hook-ups by wrapping lines and leaders in the maze of dead branches under that big tree.

Miraculously, the fish came out and plowed toward the middle of the river, but he never made it. He was fighting both the current and all the pressure I dared put on my 10-pound test tippet. Shortly, he tired, but not before I slipped off a sloping rock and dunked myself and my camera in the swift water. I held on and was finally able to bring him to net.

My wet camera provided a rather poor picture, but my Zebco De-Liar said the big fish weighed five pounds and measured 23 inches in length, a chunky male and my largest trout ever from all my years of angling in Yellowstone country. After I carefully revived him in shallow water, I released him back into the river.

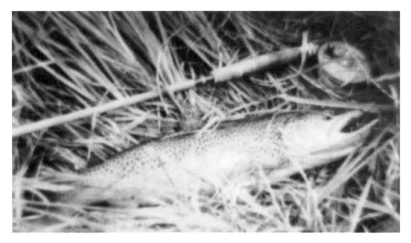

A poor picture caused by the dunking my camera and I took while fighting this five-pound, 23-inch brown trout in the Madison River

WHEN RICK AND I rendezvoused later that day, I enjoyed telling him "the rest of the story" as radio's Paul Harvey used to say. And when we got back to Clemson, I bought a waterproof camera.

At another time on this trip to Yellowstone, Rick and I hiked down a very small stream named DeLacy Creek that feeds into Shoshone Lake. The creek was loaded with Eastern brook trout that had been stocked in the park in the early decades of the 20th century. Rick and I were hoping that some of the large brown trout in the lake were swimming up the little creek to spawn.

Unfortunately, we were about a month too early for those spawners, but brookies were so plentiful that it was hard to keep them off the hook. On one single cast I caught two small brookies on a #16 elk-hair caddis, the only time I have ever done that!

Rick said he caught a 12-inch brookie, a really nice brookie from such a small creek, but I didn't see it so I can't verify his story! Ha,ha,

Rick! He also claimed to have caught more trout than I did. Again, I didn't see all the fish he claimed to have caught, so he may have been exaggerating a little bit, as fishermen are prone to do.

Then and now, we'll still kid each other about who had the largest catch on this trip into DeLacy Creek. It's all in good fun. We don't lie — at least not much — about anything as serious as fishing. But I did have photographic proof of two small brookies on one cast. Rick couldn't match that!

Chapter 17

Other Memorable Trips to the Rockies

SOMETIMES, CAROLYN AND I drove south from Yellowstone to the Grand Tetons National Park in Wyoming, where, over the decades, I occasionally fished the Snake, Gros Ventre and Hoback rivers. Twice I fished Flat Creek, a quiet meadow stream just north of Jackson, Wyoming, that flows gently through the National Elk Refuge. On my first trip there in early August of 2008, the mosquitos almost "ate me alive," but I was able to catch a few cutthroats before the bloodthirsty insects ran me off the stream.

On my second trip in late September 2009, the cutthroats, supposedly one of the easiest trout to catch, taught me a lesson in humility. The months of August and September had been dry in the Yellowstone-Grand Teton ecosystem. That was a good sign, I thought, because without standing water in the flat meadows around the stream, mosquitos would not be bothersome on this day.

However, the clerk at Jack Dennis's fly shop in Jackson, where I had stopped to get some inside information and buy a few flies, told me that the trout in Flat Creek had been pounded hard that summer and had become quite selective, meaning they would not eat just any old fly. Your fly had to be a close representation of what they were feeding on. These cutthroats were not going to be the easily caught salmonids that I was accustomed to catching.

When I pulled into the fisherman's access parking area the next morning, there were no other cars there. Good for me, I thought. I never like to feel pressured by other fishermen.

The young clerk at the fly shop was right. The fishing was tough, really tough. I fished for two hours without seeing any signs of a fish, then fished another hour with fish rising all around me, including one at least 20 inches long, but I couldn't buy a strike. I changed flies about five times, trying to find a pattern they would eat, but to no avail. This time I left Flat Creek without catching a fish. Sometimes you just have to pay your dues!

Then finally, the opportunity to fish in Canada came again!

In 2004, I returned to Alberta, this time to Edmonton, for a joint meeting of the Society of American Foresters and its Canadian counterparts, and another chance to fish the Bow River that I had fished ten years before with my graduate student, Kyle Burrell. This time Carolyn and I were there in late September, a perfect time to catch some of the river's large rainbows. I again called on Mike Guinn to be my guide.

This second trip to the Bow was my best day ever for catching large rainbow trout. Even though the river is also famous for large brown trout, I only caught one brown trout, 20-inches long. Mike explained that the browns were spawning upstream of the river section we were fishing. On this magical day, I caught and released eight large rainbows ranging from 18 to 23 inches and 15 to 20 smaller rainbows. Mike said the 23 incher, which he measured, would weigh five pounds and the two 21 inchers would weigh four pounds. What a day of fishing that was!

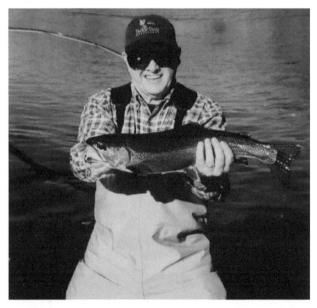

A Bow River "bullet," a 23-inch, 5-pound rainbow trout

I ALSO FISHED THE Elk River just south of Fernie, British Columbia, about 500 miles north of Yellowstone. It was a quick trip. A snowstorm was fast approaching when Carolyn and I parked by the stream. I did manage to catch and release a nice bull trout, an endangered and threatened salmonid, which is an apex predator in very cold, clear streams of the northwestern United States and western Canada. My catch was about 22 inches long, the only specimen of that species I have ever caught. I wish I had hired a guide on that trip.

I have usually found that money spent on a guide who is familiar with his local waters is money well spent.

Chapter 18

Fishing Nearer Home

SINCE THE ROCKIES ARE thousands of miles from my home in Clemson, South Carolina, I could not go there every time I needed a fly-fishing fix. So, I fished for trout in the Southern Appalachians, whose streams are underrated by many fly fishermen, but not by me. I love the swift, rocky creeks and rivers of the southern mountains and the forest vegetation of their riparian zones. Fly fishing in these streams helped me avoid feeling burned out from the daily grind of work, which, while I enjoyed it, was tiring at the pace I engaged in it.

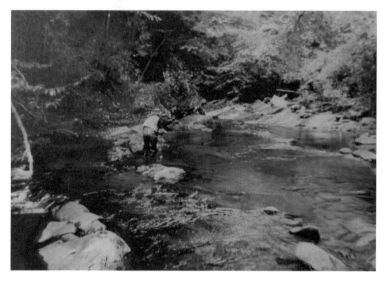

Streams in the Southern Appalachians can provide
great fishing, too.

MY FISHING JOURNALS SHOW that I frequently fished the Chattooga River, the East Fork of the Chattooga, the Whitewater, the Thompson, the Chauga, the Savannah River tailwater trout fishery and other South Carolina streams, all within about an hour's drive from Clemson.

When time allowed, I fished the Davidson River and a small tributary called Looking Glass Creek in North Carolina, plus a trophy stream called Bullpen Creek, where trout were fed several times each week by park rangers and grew ridiculously large. My largest trout from that creek was a male brown with a menacing kype, a fish that measured 25-inches long and weighed an estimated six pounds. I caught it in late April 1988 on a wooly bugger, during one of numerous trips I made to Bullpen Creek that spring, a time that was the busiest of my career. Again, fly fishing had come to my rescue.

In those days, if I couldn't talk one of my buddies into fishing with me, I would fish alone on Southern Appalachian streams. I tried to fish the best trout streams in Georgia, North Carolina, Tennessee and Virginia as often as possible. Other times from the early 1970s through 2005, I fished streams in the Great Smokies Mountains National Park. Abrams Creek and Little River were two of my favorite waters there.

I had been a chaired professor at Clemson since about 1980, an honor which carried with it certain expectations. Because I didn't want people to think I wasn't serious about my academic responsibilities, I didn't tell most people at work about my fishing habits. After all, I didn't know anyone at the university who had fishing fever as bad as I did.

Even when my wife Carolyn and I wanted to take a minivacation as we called them, it would involve fishing. We often would head for one of the streams in our neighboring states for a long weekend. We liked to stay in Townsend or Gatlinburg, Tennessee; or Dahlonega, Georgia; or Cherokee or Brevard, North Carolina, because I could fish nearby streams and Carolyn could shop or explore these quaint little towns.

I also fly fished in South Carolina's beautiful mountain lakes. In the winter of 2006-07, my good friend John Garton and I had made numerous trips from Clemson to fish Lake Jocassee. The Department of Natural Resources annually stocked this gorgeous lake with sub-legal trout, that is trout less than 15-inches long. John and I had caught and released our share during our trips to the lake. We knew there were holdover trout in the lake that were much bigger, but they were hard to catch, at least for us.

One December morning, we were fishing a cove beside one of Jocassee's boat ramps where I saw some schools of brown minnows, about an inch long, swimming close to the bank just under the surface. Then I noticed some of the recently stocked trout striking something on the surface. Maybe they were striking those minnows because we didn't see any flies hatching. The closest fly match I could think of to those small minnows was an elk-hair caddis, a dry fly which normally floats, but I manicured it with my snippers to make it sparse and slightly sinkable. The fly was now about the same size and color as those minnows, and I could swim it at about the same depth as the minnows.

I cast the fly into the middle of the cove where I had seen fish striking near the surface. Stripping the fly back, I had a hard strike. This fish was much bigger than the stocked trout that had recently been put in the lake, and it headed out to the main body of the lake, jumping three times. At last I was able to turn it and fight it back into the cove and finally into my net. It was a beautiful four-pound rainbow trout, which I released after John took a picture.

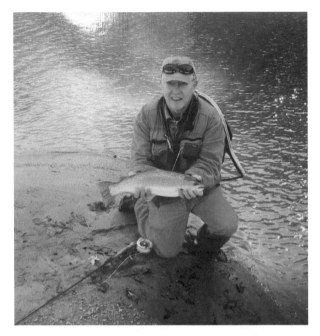

A fat, four-pound rainbow trout from Lake Jocassee,
caught on a manicured elk-hair caddis

A FEW TRIPS LATER, on January 4, John scored one of those big fish himself, catching a three- to four-pound brown, whose stomach was so distended that it looked like it was pregnant. I suspect it had been eating those minnows I had seen earlier.

On occasion, I was able to fish stocked trout ponds in the mountains of South Carolina, where trout grew large from artificial feeding. Most trout streams and ponds in South Carolina have low fertility and cannot support a large biomass (weight) of fish. However, when trout in these waters are artificially fed high-protein pellets, they can grow to be very large. They were fun to catch but didn't fulfill my urge to catch wild trout.

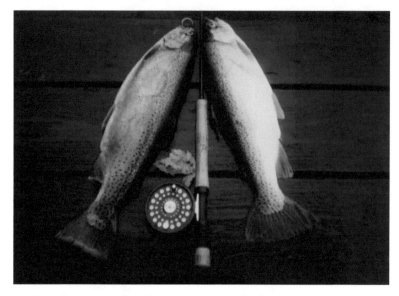

Two, four-pound rainbow trout I caught from a private pond
in the mountains of South Carolina

Chapter 19

Trout Unlimited and Giving Back

WHEN I REFLECTED ON all the memories and happiness that fly fishing had given me, I realized that I wanted to give something back to the sport. Joining Trout Unlimited (TU), a non-profit organization dedicated to the conservation of rivers and streams and their habitats for trout and salmon, back in the early 1970s was a first step in that direction. In 1988, our newly formed Chattooga River Chapter of TU asked me to lead its efforts in a partnership of federal and state agencies and conservation groups to restore trout habitat in Corbin Creek, a small stream on Duke Power, now Duke Energy, property in the mountains of South Carolina.

Our chapter installed over 40 stream improvement structures made of logs and rebar in Corbin Creek to improve trout habitat. Five to 10 of us worked many Saturdays for several years installing those structures, using chainsaws, sledgehammers and rebar, as directed by Monte Seehorn, trout biologist with the U.S. Forest Service, to provide cover and spawning habitat for trout. We cleared brush to make the stream more accessible for electrofishing and helped with fish surveys done by the South Carolina Department of Natural Resources (SCDNR).

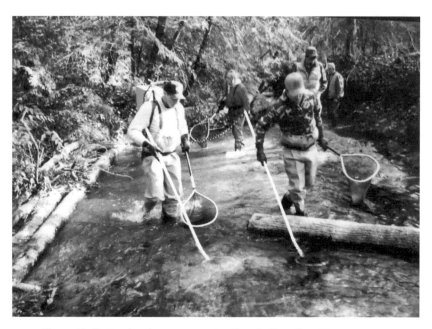

Trout Unlimited volunteers assist South Carolina Department of Natural Resources staff in electrofishing Corbin Creek. The cover logs and deflector logs are stream improvement structures that TU installed.

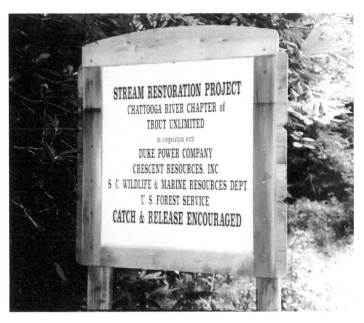

Partners on Corbin Creek restoration project

I SERVED AS THE TU project leader in a joint partnership project formed by Trout Unlimited, SCDNR, U.S. Forest Service, Duke Power and others, to restore the Southern Appalachian strain of the eastern brook trout to King Creek in 2004 and Crane Creek in 2006. Both are small headwater streams on the Sumter National Forest in South Carolina. This strain of brook trout is a genetically distinct strain that is native to the Southern Appalachian Mountains and one of the most beautiful fish you will ever see.

Although I had a heavy teaching and research load at the time, I jumped at the opportunity to lead TU's efforts on both of these projects. In this partnership, our chapter assisted the SCDNR in evaluating stream habitat and removing non-native species (brown and rainbow trout, and mixed-strain brookies) from streams selected for restoration. Then we helped stock the pure-strain brookies by toting them in oxygenated bags into distant sections of streams the DNR had deemed as suitable habitat for them.

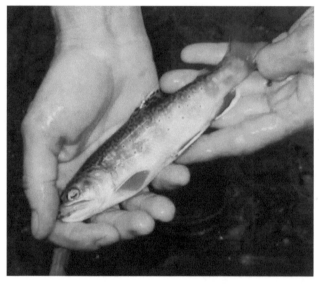

The Southern Appalachian strain of the eastern brook trout

THE PURE-STRAIN BROOKIES HAD been collected by fishery biologists from remote streams in South Carolina, North Carolina and Georgia. DNA analysis was used to ensure that these collected fish were the pure strain before stocking them in streams where non-native species and hybrids had been removed. Subsequent surveys in the following years showed that the pure-strain brookies we helped stock were reproducing, indicating that restoration efforts were successful.

When I completed my participation on these projects in 2009, it was time for me to retire from leading some of the chapter's projects.

I had worked for over two decades, from 1988 to 2009, as our chapter's lead person on several of its trout conservation and restoration projects. Now I felt that I had given enough back to the sport that had meant so much to me. It was a good feeling, for sure.

Chapter 20

Accomplishments at Clemson

I RETIRED FROM CLEMSON when I turned 65. I had grown weary, after 35 years, of preparing lectures, grading tests, writing and editing papers, theses and dissertations, going to meetings and serving on many university and graduate-student committees.

When I retired, I had been well rewarded for my accomplishments, probably more so than I deserved. While I like to believe my colleagues thought of me as a very modest and humble guy, I'll admit that an elevated self-esteem is yet one more symptom of cyclothymia! I would never brag out loud to anyone about my accomplishments, although I did hang my plaques and awards on my office wall at the request of my department head.

In 1980, I was named a chaired professor at Clemson — the Robert Adger Bowen Professor of Forest Resources. I was recognized by the Society of American Foresters (SAF) for leading a task force in writing "Choices in Silviculture for American Forests" in 1981 and was elected a Fellow in SAF in 1985.

Along with my student Patrick Brose, I received the Outstanding Hardwood Researcher Award from the National Hardwood Lumber Association in 1998 and in 2001, I was named the Outstanding Alumnus of the College of Forest Resources at Virginia Tech. I received the Godley-Snell Award for excellence in Agricultural Research at Clemson in 2002. In 2003, the South Carolina Forestry Association presented me with the Charles Flory Award for distinguished service. In 2003, SAF honored me with the Barrington Moore Memorial Award for distinguished biological research.

The Clemson Chapter of Sigma Xi named me Researcher of the Year in 2005 and, in the same year, the Association of Fire Ecology presented me with a lifetime achievement award. All of these awards were based primarily on my research accomplishments, none of which would have been possible without my graduate students, technicians and peers who cooperated with me.

I also received awards from the university and SAF for teaching and advising student organizations. Under my guidance as adviser, the Clemson Student Chapter received the national SAF Outstanding Student Chapter Award, in 1997-98 and 1998-99.

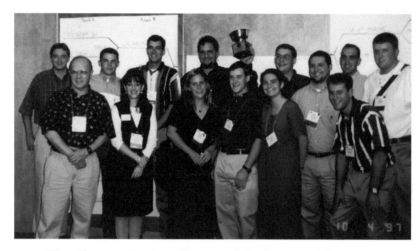

The Clemson Student Chapter of the Society of American Foresters twice won Outstanding Student Chapter in the Nation awards while I was adviser.

TROUT UNLIMITED PRESENTED ME with a Distinguished Service Award in 2010 for my efforts in leading its stream and brook trout restoration efforts in South Carolina.

Chapter 21

Retirement and Beyond

BEING A PRODUCTIVE PROFESSOR was rewarding, but can be exhausting, and it was time for me to hang it up, as far as the academic life was concerned. Now, I wanted to spend more time with my wife, who I love dearly.

I also had become hesitant about fishing the slippery, rocky and swift trout streams of the Southern Appalachians and Rocky Mountains. When I was a younger man, I took a couple of nasty falls hopping from slippery rock to slippery rock in trout streams or jumping off the bow of my boat onto rocky rip-rap, missing the rock and falling, as the boat drifted away from the ramp (as witnessed by my friend Willy who was with me that day).

While I knew this was craziness when I got into my 60s, I couldn't give up fishing altogether. It's hard to give up an addiction. Instead, I began to fish small ponds near Clemson for bluegills, redbreast and largemouth bass — a much safer venture for an old codger.

Luckily, there are numerous farm ponds and old river channels that have been impounded near Clemson. Some are on campus and on the university's extended campus, the Clemson Experimental Forest, which contains Lake Issaqueena, a 150-acre lake that feeds into Lake Hartwell. Nearly all of these impoundments have good populations of panfish and largemouth bass.

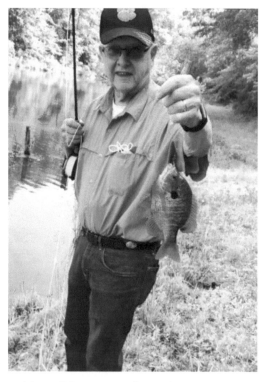

A bluegill from a small pond near Clemson

SWITCHING MY FISHING TO lakes and ponds didn't mean there were no more adventures. Near the end of my fishing journal entries, I see one, in March 2009, that is memorable, not only because of the fishing but because it nearly cost me my life. I have had too many close calls!

On this day, I was fishing again with Kyle Burrell, my former graduate student who had become a fishing guide. We had been fishing the Chattahoochee River that flows through Atlanta, a river that was first stocked with trout in 1962, possible because of cold flows from the depths of Lake Lanier upstream. Kyle guides on the Chattahoochee during the winter, and I was fortunate to be able to book him for this trip.

We had a very good day. Kyle kept track of the fish I caught and counted 36, ranging from nine to 14 inches. No big ones, but we had a lot of fun.

Then I started back to Clemson. I had recently found out that I had diabetes, and my blood sugar had been fluctuating like crazy. What I did not know at the time was that when my sugar was dropping rapidly, I would get very sleepy.

About halfway home from Atlanta, I became aware that I was having a hard time staying awake. Of course, I should have pulled over and taken a nap or eaten a sugary snack, but I didn't, and I fell asleep at the wheel. There I was, driving in the left lane of the extremely busy Interstate 85, going north at 70 mph, when suddenly I felt and heard a loud thump on the passenger side of my pickup.

I had drifted into the trailer of a big truck that was in the right lane! The thump I felt was my passenger-side mirror colliding with the metal strip at the bottom of the semi-trailer, right in front of its back wheels. The impact folded my mirror flat against the window.

Talk about a wake up! Miraculously, I was able to maintain control of my truck after the mini-collision, and the driver of the heavy tractor trailer probably never even realized I had run into him. What a close call! If I had been driving my Camry, which I considered driving that morning and which sits much lower on the road, I would have drifted under that semi-trailer and certainly been crushed and killed.

That day, still shaking, I pulled off at the next rest stop, to straighten my mirror and try to calm myself down. The only damage to my truck was a scratch on my right mirror where it hit the semi. I had learned a lesson, and after this incident, I got my diabetes under reasonable control with medication and exercise. "Good thinking, Dave," I told myself. "It only took a near-death experience to get you to act."

I am not sure why I have been so lucky in my life, but I am thankful for my blessings.

I have had many friends over my lifetime, including some who over years and years have become really special. One is John Garton, who with his wife Kathy, also lives at Clemson Downs where Carolyn and I now live. When the weather is favorable, John and I frequently meet at a swing overlooking a beautiful view of the Downs campus, where we reminisce about our friendship and fishing memories over the past 40 years. Sometimes Clemson football finds its way into our conversation. The overlook is a quiet place, and we can both hear each other, especially when I snap my speaker microphone to his shirt.

John and I are so compatible because we come from similar life experiences. Both of us began fishing at a young age for smallmouth bass in clear, cool-water streams, he on Mill Creek in Tennessee and me on the Cowpasture River in Virginia. We both studied natural resource fields in college. John holds a B.S. in wildlife management and a M.S. in biology from Tennessee Tech, a good match for my B.S. and M.S. in forest management and Ph.D. in forest sciences.

We first became really close friends because of our efforts in conservation. In 1976, we met on a field trip into the Whitewater River watershed to observe the conservation measures put in place by Duke Energy to minimize erosion during construction of the Bad Creek hydro project, a pump storage facility used to generate electricity during peak demand periods. John was a wildlife biologist for Duke Energy, and I was an associate professor of forestry at Clemson, but I was representing Trout Unlimited on this field trip.

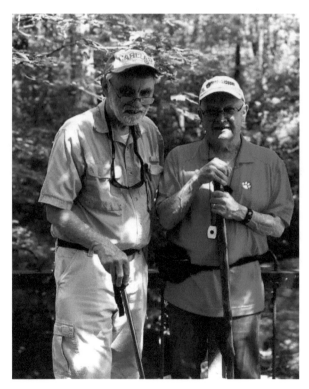

My friend of forty plus years, John Garton, and me

JOHN LED A PARTNERSHIP of conservation groups, academics and Duke Energy employees in developing a plan to protect the White-water River, one of only a few pristine trout streams in South Carolina. We were both members of Trout Unlimited and, over the next 25 years, worked on several conservation projects together, including the improvement of trout habitat in Corbin Creek.

We both led TU's efforts in helping restore the Southern Appalachian strain of the eastern brook trout to several small headwater streams in the mountains of South Carolina, and we have served as board members of the South Carolina Wildlife Federation (SCWF) in which John had played a major role for many years. The SCWF partnered on numerous conservation projects we undertook.

John and I led field trips and camping trips for TU and SCWF during the 1990s. On one field trip we led to the Clemson Experimental Forest, at a stop overlooking Issaqueena Lake, a majestic bald eagle flew by in full view for the entire length of the 150-acre lake. I had only seen one other bald eagle in the experimental forest in 30 years. What a way to spice up a field trip for two naturalists!

Another longtime friend, Rick Myers, came into my life as one of my undergraduate students back in the late 1970s. Rick was not only a very good student, he was also a fisherman. That helped cement our friendship.

The first time I became aware of Rick as a fisherman was when my friend Willy Williams and I encountered Rick and Jud Alden, then undergraduates, along the West Fork of the Chattooga River, a remote stream in northeastern Georgia. It is a long-distance hike to get to the river and the elevation difference between the parking area and the river is at least 1,000 feet — it seems like more, especially when hiking out. I knew right then that Rick was a good man and so was Jud. They became two of my favorite graduate students.

After Rick completed his Bachelor of Science in forestry, he stayed at Clemson University for his Master of Science working with Dr. Bob Zahner. Then he went to work for Purdue University as manager of the school's forest.

Prior to beginning his Ph.D. program, Rick and I took annual leave from Clemson in mid-September 1986 and went to Yellowstone National Park for a week of trout fishing. We needed a break. That turned out to be one of the best weeks of trout fishing I have ever had. We fished most of the famous streams inside and just outside of the park, including the Gallatin, Madison, Lamar and Yellowstone rivers, plus two smaller creeks, Iron Creek and DeLacy Creek.

We had great fishing every day, but a few days stand out. One was the day I caught the biggest brown trout I ever caught in Yellowstone country, a hook-jawed male that was 23 inches long and weighed five pounds. Finally, I had caught a brown trout a little bigger than my old friend Richard Deeds' four pounder from Iron Creek in 1958. It only took me 28 years to do it! When I wrote about our hike to the Yellowstone River in my fishing journal, I recorded that I saw a grizzly bear two- to three-hundred yards up the mountain, above the river, foraging in an open meadow. We had hiked four miles to the river, following Blacktail Deer Creek all the way, and had seen bear warning signs at several places along the trail. I still had the jitters about seeing grizzly bears, ever since I was treed by a mother grizzly with cubs in 1961. And that darned Rick kept singing a grizzly bear song all the way to the river, just to keep me on edge!

On this day, as soon as I saw the grizzly, I immediately crossed the footbridge to put the river between me and the bear. I tried calling out a warning to Rick who was still on the grizzly side of the river, but the river's roar prevented him from hearing me. Thankfully, Rick soon followed me and crossed the river to the "safe" side.

When Hurricane Hugo hit South Carolina's coast in 1989, I received a grant from the U.S. Forest Service to study the response of forest vegetation to the visibly extreme damage caused by the hurricane. I knew that hurricanes had been impacting the South Carolina coast for millennia and that native Americans would have set fires to clear the debris on these hurricane-impacted landscapes to enable them to maneuver, hunt and survive. The U.S. Forest Service wanted to know how forested coastal ecosystems respond to these types of historical disturbances.

Because I needed a Ph.D. student to take the lead on the project, I contacted Rick to see if he would be interested. He agreed to come back to Clemson and did a fine job on the project.

Thirty years later, it was Rick and Jud, who invited me to Virginia to fish the Calfpasture River for a trip that rejuvenated me, making me look forward to the next ten years of my life.

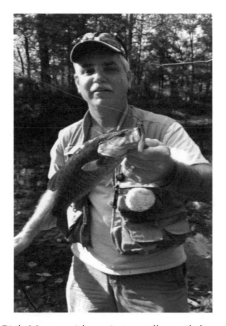

Rick Myers with a nice smallmouth bass
from the Calfpasture River

Chapter 22

My Lifelong Love and Living at the Downs

WHEN I LIST THE great loves of my life, I must start with Carolyn. Forty-three years after our first meeting, Carolyn is still the love of my life. She is the only woman I have ever really been in love with, and she has been my best friend, too. Carolyn didn't fish, although I tried to teach her the basics. However, Carolyn was my frequent companion when I traveled to professional meetings all over the country, in Canada and even to Europe. She even tolerated the many times I would escape for a few days of fishing before or after my meetings. While I fished, she would entertain herself by reading, doing needlepoint, or shopping. When we took minivacations, she loved the company of our dog, or dogs, who stayed with her and "guarded" her while I fished.

Carolyn was so tolerant of my need to fish. While most wives would probably have divorced me, Carolyn understood and never complained one time. She never criticized me when I was feeling down or trying to do too much; she just offered support. To me, she is the prettiest, sweetest and most tolerant woman I have ever known. I was so blessed to have married her.

When Carolyn and I married, I was accepted into my new family fairly well, although it took the children, especially Melanie, a while to get used to me. I had always wanted to have a wife and a son and daughter, the perfect family. In a freshman English class at Hampden-Sydney in 1958, a professor had asked us to write an essay about our aspirations. I said my long-term aspirations were to get married and have a family. It only took me 20 years to accomplish that dream. Better late than never, they say!

This situation seemed ideal; I had a beautiful and loving wife, two children, both of whom were beyond the diaper stage (which I'm not sure I could have handled). I soon learned that being a stepparent is not the easiest job in the world. I wanted to be a good father to both children, and I believe they both came to love me.

I dreamed of teaching Chris to fish, maybe even to fly fish, but he did not catch the fishing bug. I took him fishing a few times, but he was more interested in cars and engineering than in the outdoors and fishing. I was disappointed but accepted his lack of interest.

Melanie, however, was wired the opposite way. She was very artistic but, to my way of thinking, not very logical. She could be very sweet but was moody, at times hard to live with. Of course, that might have been me, not her. Melanie made me realize that being a stepdad was tough, really tough.

Yet even when my dreams and reality didn't match up, I was very happy with my situation.

Chris made the decision to go to Clemson University and major in mechanical engineering. He did very well, graduated on time and accepted a job with Honeywell in Florida. Chris has remained a bachelor, happy with his single life.

During her senior year of high school, Melanie attended the North Carolina School of the Arts in Winston-Salem. She graduated from there, a very talented visual artist.

One of the secrets to 43 years of happy marriage for Carolyn and me has been our willingness to compromise and avoid being dogmatic on our differing positions. Our love has been so true that we couldn't bear the thought of making the other partner feel sad or depressed because of a silly argument. Consequently, we hardly ever argued and if we did, we did it with civility.

Another of the secrets to our long-lasting marriage was that we liked so many of the same things, like eating out at restaurants, country music and country music shows, traveling in the Rocky Mountains and Southern Appalachians, Clemson sports, our dogs and loving our children. There weren't many things we disagreed on, so there was no reason to argue.

Over these 40-plus years, she has been a great mother and was a wonderful daughter to her aging parents — just a darned good person.

In our retirement years, Carolyn and I enjoyed camping in the Southern Appalachians in our camper. Our dogs, first Ginger, then Cricket and Dolly, and finally just Dolly, would go with us and keep Carolyn company while I would fish. Our dogs were so much a part of our lives, and we treated them like they were our children.

About nine years ago, Carolyn and I moved into Clemson Downs, a retirement community. We wanted to make the move before we got too "old and decrepit."

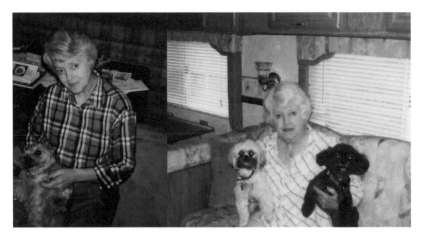

Carolyn with Ginger, and Carolyn in our camper
with Cricket and Dolly

CLEMSON DOWNS HAS BEEN a wonderful place for us. It has a beautiful campus, great administration and staff, sweet nursing assistants who bring our medicines and many activities for residents to participate in.

Moving here was a great decision because just a few years after the move, we both started having health problems. About four years ago, Carolyn had to move from our independent living apartment to health care. She had begun having minor memory problems and hygiene issues. I was growing deafer by the year, a problem I inherited from my mom's side of the family. Because of my deafness, I had quit driving, so I couldn't drive us to appointments.

When I turned 70, I had a series of serious health issues, all of which required surgery. First, I had kidney cancer that required removal of my left kidney — thankfully humans have two of those, and I recovered completely from that operation. Then, just a few years later, I had brain surgery to correct a balance and falling problem caused by what doctors diagnosed as normal pressure hydroceph-alus — in layman's terms, excess water (cerebrospinal fluid) on the brain. And finally, two years after that, I had surgery to remove a painful spur on my spine that doctors thought was causing me to be bent over at the waist and walk with a cane.

I soon realized Carolyn and I needed a caregiver to help take care of us and drive us to appointments.

Luckily, the head nurse here at Clemson Downs knew of a woman who had worked as a caregiver for almost two decades and was now looking for another client. That would be us!

Diane Blackmon has been a godsend for us.

Diane's entrance into our lives was a major turning point in my life and Carolyn's as well. And she came at a time I didn't think there would be any more turning points. She changed my attitude about Clemson Downs as a friend says, "from being a place to die to being a place to live."

Diane is loyal and caring, as well as being extremely smart and multi-talented for sure. Soon after she started working for us, she had to rush me to the emergency room because my blood potassi-um levels had risen to dangerous levels. The doctor thought I was in danger of having a heart attack. Diane not only drove me to the hospital, but she stayed with me for 14 hours in the emergency room until my potassium returned to normal levels. How many caregivers would do that?

Diane does our laundry, cleans our apartment, drives us wherever and whenever we need to go, keeps track of all our appointments and is the liaison with our lawyer and accountant. She is also a sounding board for our children and has a great sense of humor, which Caro-lyn and I love. Diane does so much more than the average caregiver, and she does it willingly and with an Alabama drawl that makes her English unique and special. Diane seems to be able to do everything, from repairing my furniture to decorating my apartment. She once even re-built a Harley-Davidson motorcycle for herself. And yes, she used to be a Harley girl, claims she still is. Diane is also our psychologist who listens not only to Carolyn and me but our children, as well. Thank goodness she doesn't charge what psychologists do!

Diane loves dogs, and they love her. Before Carolyn went to health care, where she gets round-the-clock care, Diane would take us to breakfast and dinner frequently. When she would take me out to meals, before the Covid-19 pandemic, we would take Dolly, our little 6½-pound shih-tzu, weather permitting. Dolly, who we had to put down when she was nearly 17 years old, thought she was a big guard dog as she sat on the center console between the front seats of Diane's car and kept watch while we are eating, even though she couldn't see much anymore.

We all look forward to the end of the virus scare when we can all go out to eat again, this time with Tiger, our new little shih tzu, as the guard dog.

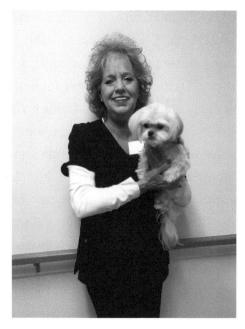

Our caregiver, Diane Blackmon, and Dolly

DIANE CAN BE A little "bossy," which is exactly what I needed. When Diane arrived, I needed someone to encourage me, in fact, order me, to get up and get on with my life. Without her encouragement, I wouldn't have made the amazing physical and mental recovery that I have made over the last couple of years.

Diane has cared for others, too. She raised her grandson from the time he was just four years old. Now he is a sergeant in the U.S. Marines who adores her, as Carolyn and I do.

Diane, to me, is a great person who came into our life when we needed her and has become like a daughter to us.

Thanks to Diane and other caregivers and friends, Carolyn and I move forward. Carolyn's memory struggle has been hard, but her long-term memory is remarkable. Because of the Covid-19 virus in

2020 and 2021, the health-care area of Clemson Downs has been under lockdown. I cannot physically touch and hug her, but I can see her through a glass window. When I was talking to her via phone during one of our recent closed-window visits, she suddenly asked me, "Are the Craighead brothers still alive?"

What??

The Craigheads were grizzly-bear researchers in Yellowstone Park back in the 1960s and 1970s, more than 50 years ago. I don't know how Carolyn made that connection after so many years, except that the memory must have been burned into her mind from a film about the Craigheads we saw in the museum in West Yellowstone.

I, too, struggle with being nearly deaf in the age of Covid-19, when everybody is, or should be, wearing a mask. First, the mask muffles slightly the voice of the speaker, making it harder for them to be understood. And second, I cannot read lips when the speaker is wearing a mask. I was never a very good lip reader, but I was good enough that seeing the lips move helped a little bit.

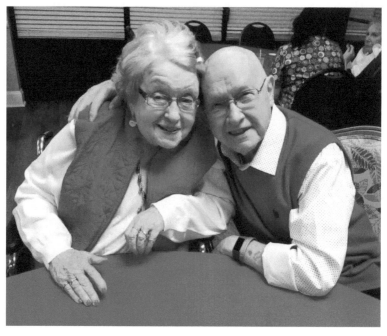

Carolyn and me celebrating Christmas 2021
at Clemson Downs

YET THESE DAYS I consider myself fortunate to have made some re-markable comebacks. After three surgeries, at age 70 my health was still in decline. I was still bent over, and the pain in my back was so bad and my balance so poor that I bought a motor scooter to get me around the Downs campus. I couldn't walk the 50 yards to the dining hall without almost falling, and occasionally I did. This time my problem was diagnosed as inflamed arthritis and a slipped disc in my spine.

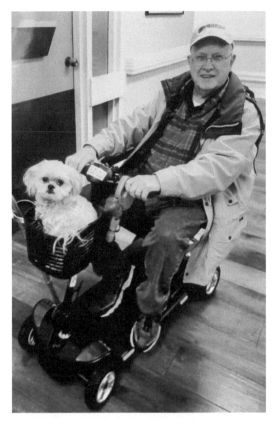

Dolly and me on my scooter in 2018, when I could
hardly walk 50 yards without almost falling

MY BACK SURGEON WANTED to do more surgery on my spine, but I didn't want that, since the last back surgery hadn't helped me, and I was sick of surgeries. So, I asked my brain surgeon for a second opinion. She examined the X-rays and MRIs of my back and instead of suggesting more surgery, sent me to a pain management clinic in Anderson, South Carolina. There, a doctor injected steroids into my spine, a slightly uncomfortable but not too painful procedure, even for a wimp like me.

Within days, the pain in my back was almost gone, and I could stand up straight again. Because of the forceful orders of our wonderful caregiver, Diane, I began to go to an exercise class five days a week led by the Clemson Downs' dynamic exercise leader Anayeli "Ana" Olayo.

Ana has also helped to turn my life around, both physically and mentally. She has been more than my exercise leader, she is a trusted friend who, in addition, has taken me to fish in her uncle's small pond that is loaded with bluegills and some bass. Aha! Fishing to the rescue again!

I go to Ana's exercise class five times a week. Although it is called seated exercise, we do vigorous aerobics, stretching, weight training and other exercises. She especially emphasizes exercises that strengthen those core muscles located deep within your trunk which help you stand up straight. Her exercise program has worked wonders for me.

Within weeks of starting Ana's classes, I began feeling so much stronger that I began hiking with Ana and her hiking group. We began by hiking only one day a week but have gradually increased the frequency of our hiking to five days a week, weather permitting. We hike for about 30 to 45 minutes on trails and roads around Clemson Downs. Covid-19 shut down our classes temporarily, but we are now back on schedule.

I credit determination and the efforts of Diane and Ana for my most recent and enjoyable adventures.

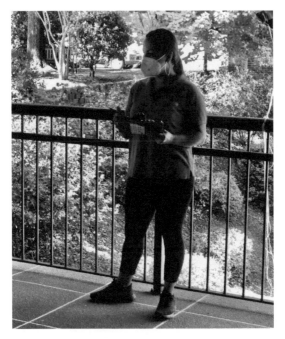

Anayeli Olayo (wearing her Covid-19 mask) is my exercise
leader who played a major role in rejuvenating me both
physically and mentally.

Chapter 23

One Last Fishing Trip, or is It?

By the time I reached 79 years old, I thought that because of my health problems and not driving anymore my fishing days were over. I had not fished seriously for almost 10 years.

But once again fishing came to the rescue.

Out of the blue, in September 2019, two of my former graduate students, Rick Myers and Jud Alden, invited me to go to Virginia and fish the Calfpasture River over the Columbus Day weekend. This was the river I had fished 65 years earlier as a teenager, and I considered this river and its big sister, the Cowpasture, to be my home waters.

Of course, my urge to fish was strong. I was convinced that fishing was in my blood. Even 10 years earlier in my book *Memories Made and Lessons Learned During a Lifetime of Angling*, I had recognized my addiction.

I initially declined because I was concerned that Carolyn would worry too much about me.

Then Diane told me in no uncertain terms that I *was* going on this fishing trip; she would take care of Carolyn and our little dog Dolly. She said I had worked too hard over the past year to improve my physical condition not to go. She thought I could withstand the rigors of walking and wading the rocky shoreline of a small Virginia river for six to seven hours which may sound like a rather easy task for a young man, but I wasn't so sure about me. After all, it was just a year ago that I had used a motorized scooter to get around, even for short distances. I had been stooped over from pain in my back and depressed from all the surgeries I had. But now, I thought, I was pretty healthy for an old codger, able to stand and walk upright for considerable distances, and my mental outlook on life was so much better.

The decision was made. I would go fishing again in a river I had fished over 60 years ago, the Calfpasture River.

It had been a long time since I seriously wet a line. Would I have the same fire for fishing? Would the Calfpasture River area, the forests, streams and wildlife, be as I remembered them? Just about everything in my world had dramatically changed over the past 60 years, often not for the better. It was hard to imagine the Calfpasture and its environment had not changed, too. I would soon find out.

The first obstacle in my mind was how to get to Rick's home in Hanover County, Virginia, about 400 miles from Clemson. I didn't drive anymore.

Rick and Jud had already solved that problem. Jud, who lives just outside Atlanta, would pick me up on the Saturday morning of Columbus Day weekend and drive me to Virginia. We would spend the night at Rick's house, get up early on Sunday and drive the three hours to the Calfpasture River.

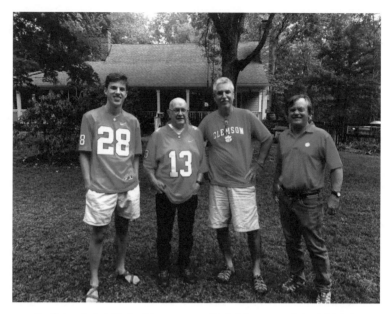

(Left to right) Cole Myers, me, Rick Myers and Jud Alden
in our Clemson shirts at Rick's house, ready to watch the
Clemson-Florida State football game

THE CALFPASTURE IS A small river, more like a creek when the water is low. Virginia had been in a severe drought during the summer of 2019 and the river was low and clear, making the fish wary and difficult to catch, more for me than for Rick, Jud and Cole, Rick's son. I started fishing with my fly rod, but my casting was pretty rusty — 10 years of absence will do that to you — and my vision so poor — 79 years of living will do that to you — that often I didn't see or connect on strikes.

I did manage to catch a few fish on my fly rod, but soon saw the wisdom of Cole's suggestion that I might catch more fish if I switched to one of their spinning outfits. That is a hard admission for a fly fisherman to make, but age will make you do strange things sometimes.

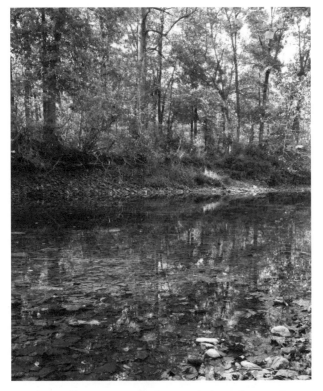

The Calfpasture River, low and clear during the
droughty summer of 2019

THANKFULLY, WITH COLE'S TUTELAGE, I began to catch fish at a faster rate. Although my numbers were not impressive, I did manage to catch what my companions called a Calfpasture Grand Slam: smallmouth bass, redeye, redbreast sunfish and fallfish.

So, I caught a grand slam, and I fell into the stream only once and that was not a hard fall, actually more of a slide into the shallow edge of the river when the bank gave way. Overall, not a bad performance for an old man who hadn't seriously fished for a decade.

The real fishermen, Rick, Jud and Cole, far out-fished me. But I enjoyed the companionship, the fishing and the beautiful environment immensely. I was fishing with two of my favorite former students from about 30 years ago, and my new friend Cole, Rick's son, had willingly consented to be my guide, possibly because I tried to teach him some of the basics of fly tying on that Saturday evening at Rick's house.

What more could I have asked for? The weather was gorgeous, the land beautiful and scarcely changed from how I remembered it long ago. Wildlife was abundant (two bald eagles, a coyote, many songbirds and lots of deer), and the river had plenty of fish. The human population density was low, there were no superhighways, no fast-food restaurants and no large urban areas, just the two small, peaceful country towns of Churchville and Deerfield. It seemed that modern society had not yet encroached on this idyllic rural environment. Here, along the Calfpasture, man and nature were in complete harmony.

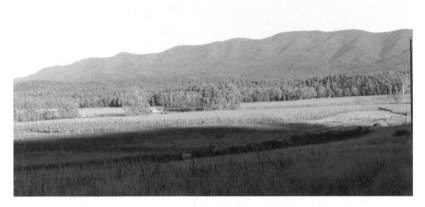

The Calfpasture River that flows through private farmland in
the Ridge and Valley province of Virginia, is today much like
it was 60 years ago.

AFTER I'D SUFFERED ALMOST a decade of serious health problems,
this trip to the Calfpasture with old friends rejuvenated me, making
me believe I could now live at least to age 90 and still fish a little bit
now and then.

Chapter 24

Fly Fishing as Philosophy

If fly fishing is as beneficial to a healthy state of mind as I claim, why don't more people do it? I believe many people have long held the impression that fly fishing is too difficult to learn. But that attitude has been gradually changing over the past couple of decades, and there are now more fly fishermen than ever, with more joining the numbers every day. Many of the new fly fishers are women.

Penn State was a pioneer in teaching fly fishing, offering courses since the 1930s. Now, many universities offer such courses. Both male and female students with good instruction soon learn that fly fishing is not so difficult. While it is challenging, it is definitely not too difficult to learn, and some students will go on to enjoy a lifetime of this "good addiction."

I sometimes wish I had begun with instructors who would have taught me the basics of fly fishing. Instead, I learned to fly fish, beginning as a teenager, by reading everything I could about the sport. I've also learned from the fishing guides I have occasionally hired, but mostly I've learned by decades of trial and error on the streams of Yellowstone National Park, the Southern Appalachians and other great trout-fishing venues.

Fly fishermen make a lot of mistakes, just as they enjoy a lot of successes. I learned a lot about fly fishing by analyzing my mistakes and trying to determine what went wrong, while looking forward to trying again.

As Ralph Waldo Emerson once said, "Life is a succession of lessons which must be lived to be understood." He wasn't talking about fishing for sure, but lessons I learned from fishing, working and living helped me understand and appreciate the person I became.

Fishing, and especially fly fishing for wild trout, worked wonders for me. And it wasn't just the actual fishing that helped, I loved everything about fly fishing, from the long, limber rods to the relatively tiny colorful flies on the end of the leader, the gorgeous environments of most trout streams, the beautifully colored trout and the rich literature about the sport. Fly fishing and the crafts it led me to are hobbies that gave me much happiness for decades during my life.

Tying flies and carving fish and fishermen helped keep me mentally engaged with the sport of fly fishing even when I was not fishing. There are thousands of artificial fly patterns and dozens of books on fly tying, at least ten of which I have owned and used. There are thousands of fly tiers, many of whom are a lot better than me, but the flies I tied were good enough to catch a lot of fish.

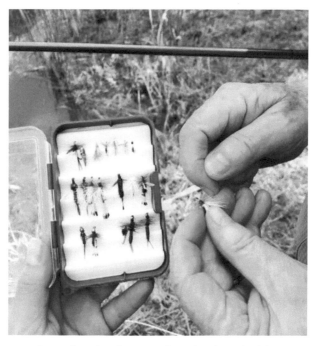

Tying flies has been a decades-long hobby

I HAD STARTED TYING flies on a rudimentary level when I was a graduate student at the University of Idaho in 1966. However, I didn't really get serious about it until I came to Clemson in 1971 and joined Trout Unlimited. Later, the officers of our newly formed Chattooga River Chapter, asked me and several others to lead classes in fly tying for our members.

I tied dozens of flies each year, mostly for my own use. My favorite flies to tie were the ones I fished with. Among the dry flies I liked to tie and fish with are: Adams, parachute Adams, elk-hair caddis, light cahills, royal coachman and thunderhead patterns. Among the nymphs and wet flies I tied and fished with were: girdle bug, peeking caddis, black gnat, prince nymph, hare's ear nymph and Montana nymph. Streamer flies I used were the dark and light spruce fly streamers and wooly buggers.

When I reached my 40s, I had become so engrossed in fly fishing that I taught myself to carve fish and fishermen from basswood or white pine. This was a hobby that came naturally to me, I think, because when I was a teenager, I had carved most of the members of a baseball team from bars of Ivory soap. I'll admit that those carved players were not works of art, but I thought they were pretty good. No one else I knew seemed able to do that. Unfortunately, sculpted bars of Ivory do not stand the test of time.

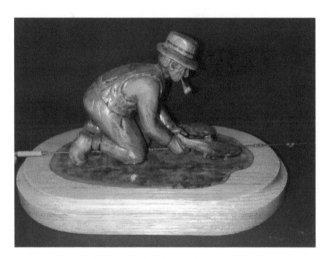

Catch and release in wood

IN MY LATE 20S, I had become an advocate of "catch and release," a term coined by Lee Wulff, a famous fly fisherman of the previous century. What could better sustain the sport of fly fishing, than for a fisherman to catch a trout and then release it to fight again another day? By doing that, another angler, or maybe even me, could catch that fish in the future. Today, many fly fishers have adopted that same culture. This way of thinking is shared by those of us in forestry, where sustainability of the resource is always on our mind.

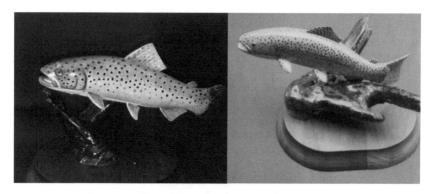

Brown and rainbow trout I carved and painted

HOWEVER, I NEVER BEGRUDGED an angler for keeping a few trout for the frying pan. I have sometimes done that myself.

So much to be grateful for

I AM SO FORTUNATE to have progressed through life to the point where I am now. I could never have dreamed when I was starting out in the mountains of Virginia (with a hillbilly accent that I didn't know I had until informed by friends working with me in Yellowstone), that I would go on to become a chaired professor at Clemson University, that I would marry the woman of my dreams and have 43 years in a happy marriage, and that I would fish some of the world's most beautiful waters with good friends. What a fairy-tail life!

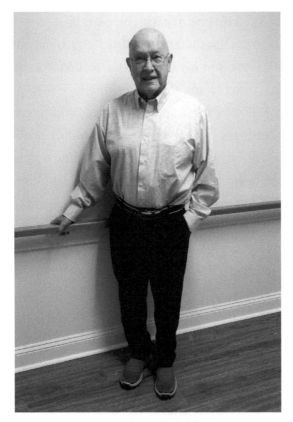

81 years old and still going strong

RECENTLY, I HAVE BEEN reflecting back on the chronology of my life, thinking about the numerous turning points that shaped the direction of my life. In particular, I've noticed how several turning points led to this life-long addiction to fishing, especially fly fishing.

I am content with my addiction.

I have ever told anyone, not even family members, that I believe I might be mildly bipolar. This is my first time to speak out. For all these years, I just kept this secret to myself and tried to use it to my advantage. But you have seen in my story the reasons I believe this to be true. I often read that people with bipolar disorder are more prone than the average person to harmful addictions, often with disastrous consequences. I saw it in my own family. Not so with fishing.

It certainly seems to me that fly fishing has been a positive addiction for me. It gave me so much pleasure and helped lift me out of occasional sadness. It enabled me to be highly productive in my field and earn many awards in research, teaching and advising. And it placed me in beautiful natural surroundings with terrific friends.

Some would say that I have been blessed, others might say I have been lucky. I am not sure which of these applies to me, maybe both, but I am grateful for a life shaped by positive turning points. It's been a wonderful one indeed.